Afsaneh Ismaili
Fatemeh Maddahi
Elahe Horri

General and Clinical Anatomy

Afsaneh Ismaili
Fatemeh Maddahi
Elahe Horri

General and Clinical Anatomy

Noor Publishing

Imprint

Any brand names and product names mentioned in this book are subject to trademark, brand or patent protection and are trademarks or registered trademarks of their respective holders. The use of brand names, product names, common names, trade names, product descriptions etc. even without a particular marking in this work is in no way to be construed to mean that such names may be regarded as unrestricted in respect of trademark and brand protection legislation and could thus be used by anyone.

Cover image: www.ingimage.com

Publisher:
Noor Publishing
is a trademark of
Dodo Books Indian Ocean Ltd., member of the OmniScriptum S.R.L Publishing group
str. A.Russo 15, of. 61, Chisinau-2068, Republic of Moldova Europe
Printed at: see last page
ISBN: 978-620-3-85948-5

General and Clinical Anatomy

By

Afsaneh Ismaili

BSc in Anesthesiology at Shahrekord Medical University, Iran

Fatemeh Maddahi

Undergraduate Student of Zanjan University and Member of the Research Committee of Abhar School of Nursing, Iran

Elahe Horri

MSc in Anatomy, Department of Anatomy, Faculty of Medicine, Molecular and Cell Biology Research Center, Mazandaran University of Medical Science, Sari, Iran

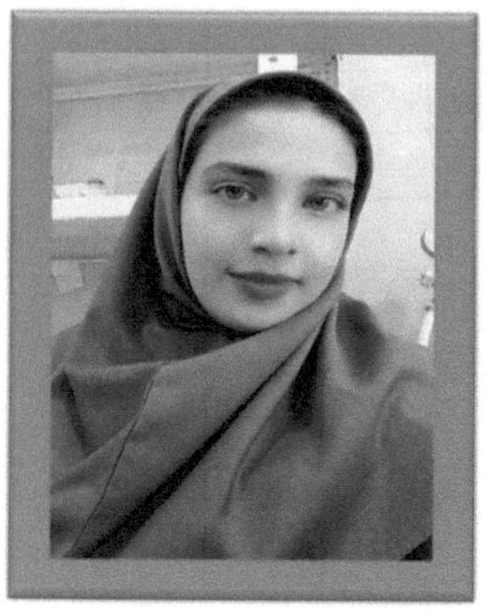

Afsaneh Ismaili

BSc in Anesthesiology at Shahrekord Medical University, Iran

Fatemeh Maddahi

Undergraduate Student of Zanjan University and Member of the
Research Committee of Abhar School of Nursing, Iran

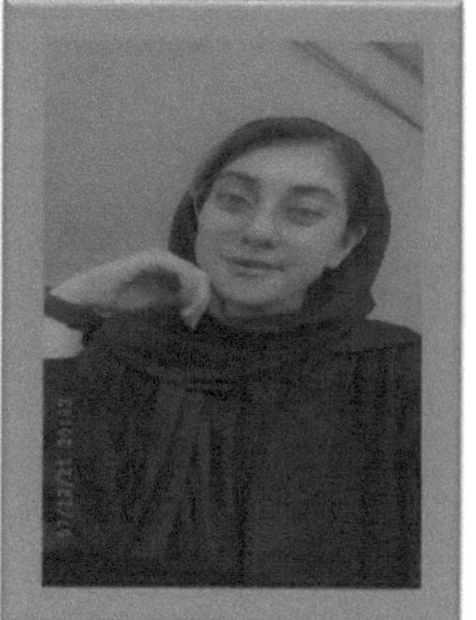

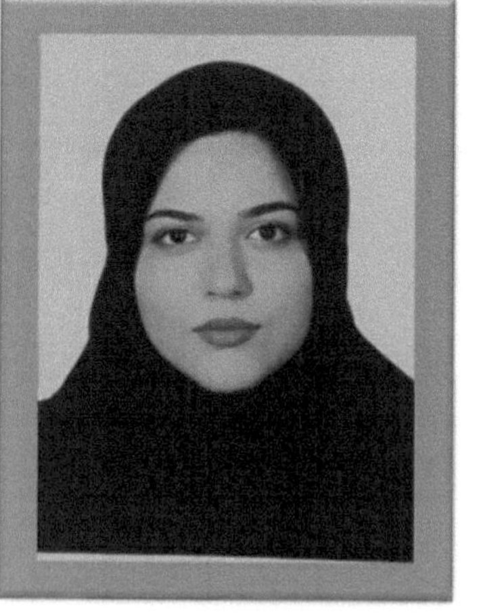

Elahe Horri

MSc in Anatomy, Department of Anatomy, Faculty of Medicine,
Molecular and Cell Biology Research Center, Mazandaran University
of Medical Science, Sari, Iran

This Book is dedicated to

My Family's

Content

Chapter I   5

Chapter II   27

Chapter III   59

Chapter IV   85

Chapter V   91

Refferences   107

Chapter I

Superficial anatomy of the back

(Surface Anatomy of the Back)

Introduction

The dorsal region extends from the skull to the end of the tailbone (Coccyx) and includes the back of the head, the back of the neck, the back of the chest, the back of the abdomen, and the upper buttocks. The back area is important because of its low back pain and spine. When examining the superficial anatomy of the back, the hands should hang loosely along the torso and the shoes should be removed.

Vertebral Column

The spine starts at the end of the skull and extends along the length of the neck and trunk. This column consists of a number of beads arranged in a row that are connected by ligaments and intervertebral discs. The length of the spine varies from person to person and the average in men is about 70 cm, which is 12 cm in the neck, 28 cm in the thoracic region, 12 cm in the lumbar region and 18 cm in the pelvic region (sacral and tail). In women, the length of the spine is 60 cm. In general, the length of the spine is two-fifths of the height of the whole body.

The length of this spine decreases in the elderly due to the decrease in the height of the intervertebral discs and the intensification of the curvature of the spine, especially the curvature of the thoracic region. The length of the spine varies around the clock and decreases by about 2 cm during the day due to its curvature. The difference in height of different people is more related to the difference in lower limb length and less to the length of the spine. The body of the third lumbar vertebra (L_3) is almost the center of the trunk in healthy people. The size of the vertebral trunk increases from the second cervical vertebra (C_2) to the third lumbar vertebra (L_3), but then decreases rapidly to the tip of the tail (Coccyx). The spine can withstand a weight of about 355 kg without breaking and a tension of 125 kg without tearing.

The weakest part of the spine is the neck area, which usually carries the least body weight, depending on how the force is applied. Most injuries occur in areas of the spine where a relatively fixed part joins a relatively moving part, such as the area where the thorax connects to the lumbar spine, or where force is applied by levers (such as the

Dens of axis and intervertebral discs), or by direct force. Such as tailbone). Fractures and dislocations of the spine depend on the location of the impact. Forced flexion is a fracture of the fifth and sixth thoracic vertebrae (T_5-T_6); Chest to second lumbar (T_9 to L_2) occurs.

The curvatures of the spine

Natural curves

During the fetal period, the fetal spine is arched and concave forward. About 3 to 9 months after birth, when the baby tilts its head back and tries to hold its head, the cervical vertebrae become convex forward, causing a secondary curvature called cervical curvature. At about 12 to 18 months, when the baby begins to walk, the vertebrae of the lumbar region become convex forward, creating another secondary curvature called lumbar curvature, but the sinus and pelvic curves (sac and tail) are the same as the embryonic and concave forward. They remain to accommodate the viscera inside the chest and pelvis. These two are called primary curvatures.

Cervical curvature

It is convex to the front and extends from the first vertebra of the neck (C1) to the second vertebra of the thorax (T2). The foremost vertebra in this curvature is the sixth vertebra of the neck (C6).

Thoracic curvature

They are concave forward and extend from the second vertebra of the thorax (T2) to the vertebra of the duodenum (T12). This curvature is due to the greater depth behind the vertebral body.

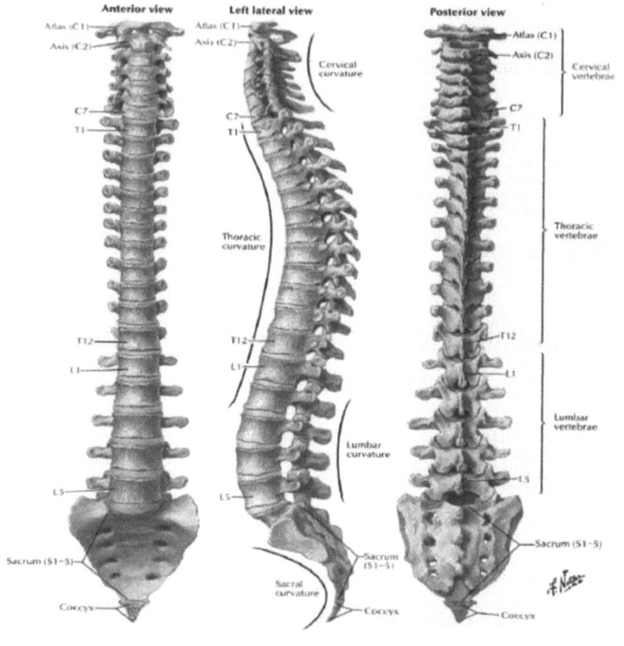

Figure 1. **Thoracic curvature**

Lumbar curvature

It is convex forward and extends from the dorsal vertebra (T12) to the joint between the fifth lumbar vertebra and the first lumbosacral joint. This curvature is due to the greater frontal depth of the disc between the vertebrae and slightly due to the shape of the vertebrae. The foremost vertebra in this curvature is the fourth lumbar vertebra (L4). This curvature is more pronounced in women.

Pelvic curvature

It is concave anteriorly and concave anteriorly (antroinferior) and extends from the lumbosacral joint to the apex of the coccyx.

Lateral curvature

In the upper chest there is a slight curvature to one side so that in right-handed people there is a slight convexity to the right of the spine and in left-handed people there is a slight convexity to the left in this area.

Natural curvature problems

The natural curvature of the vertebral column reduces the efficiency of this column as an axial skeleton. For this reason, the beads are forced to be inclined in certain areas relative to the axis of the beads. The importance of this issue becomes clear especially in the lower lumbar region, where the body of the fifth lumbar vertebra (L5) is placed on the sacrum by its intervertebral disc at an angle of 45 degrees to change the curvature of the lumbar region to the sacral region. When standing upright, the intermittent curvatures of the spine absorb direct vertical shocks. The natural curvature of this column gives it a resilient state against vertical forces so that these shocks do not enter directly into the spine, but are absorbed by the intervertebral discs and the partial bending of the curves.

The curvature of the neck is the least obvious and disappears when the neck is bent. The lumbar curvature is positioned vertically and straight, bringing the vertebral body very close to the anterior abdominal wall. It should be noted that the curves in the bony spine are more prominent and noticeable than the curves visible in the soft tissue of the trunk.

Abnormal curvatures of the spine

Kyphosis

Excessive concavity of the thoracic region is forward due to muscle weakness or structural changes in the vertebral bodies or intervertebral discs and aging. These people have a condition called Round shoulder.

Lordosis

Excessive convexity of the lumbar region is called forward as a result of weight gain on the contents of the abdomen (such as pregnancy or a large ovarian tumor) or diseases of the spine.

Scoliosis

Abnormal curvature of the spine to one side is said to occur most often in the thoracic region. Causes of this disease can be shortness of one lower limb, developmental defect of half of the body of one or both vertebrae (Hemivertebra) and paralysis of the back muscles of the spine (such as polio).

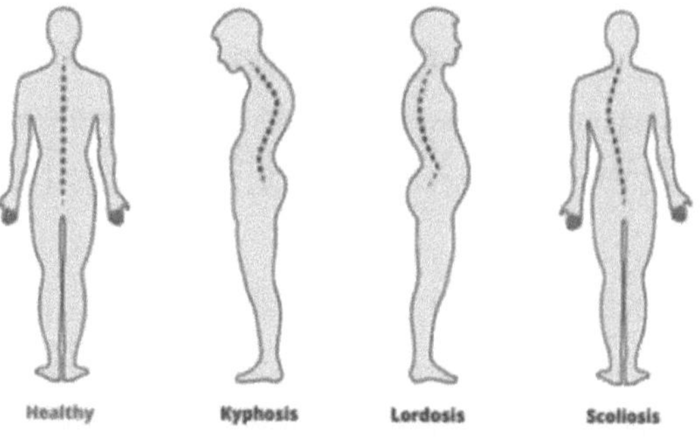

Figure 2. **Scoliosis**

Bone marks on the back

behind

External occipital protuberance

External protrusion of the back of the head is the most prominent feature of the skull, which is located at the junction of the head and neck. If we place the index finger on the scalp in the middle line and move it downwards, we will reach this protrusion along the path, which is along the Nuchal groove. The most prominent part of this area is called Inion. On each side, this linear protrusion extends to the mastoid process, known as the superior nuchal line. At the midpoint of the distance between the mammary gland and the external occipital ridge, the greater occipital nerve crosses this line and may be palpable.

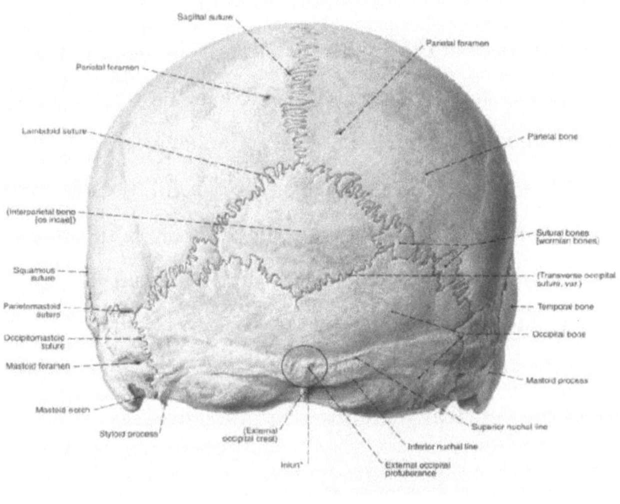

Figure 3. **External occipital protuberance**

Transverse appendages of the cervical vertebrae

The vertebrae of the cervical vertebrae are slightly more than 2.5 cm from the midline and may be felt on the skin on either side of the neck. If you connect a line from the apex of the mammary gland to the middle of the clavicle, the transverse process of the cervical vertebrae is obtained.

A) The transverse protrusion of the atlas vertebra (C1) is relatively large and can be felt approximately 1-1 / 5 cm below the apex of the mammary gland or in the distance between the mandibular angle and the mammary gland in front of the sternocleidomastoid muscle (SCM).

B) The transverse process of the second cervical vertebra (Axis) is level with the mandibular angle and deep in the SCM muscle.

C) The transverse process of the third vertebra of the neck is at the level of the upper lateral bone of the hyoid bone and deep in the SCM muscle.

D) The transverse process of the fourth cervical vertebra is flush with the upper side of the thyroid cartilage in the middle of the neck immediately behind the SCM.

E) The transverse process of the fifth vertebra of the neck is flush with the middle part of the thyroid cartilage and slightly behind the SCM muscle.

F) The transverse process of the sixth vertebra of the neck is flush with the lower side of the cricoid cartilage and can be felt in the dorsal triangle of the neck above the middle part of the clavicle. The anterior part of this transverse appendage is prominent and is known as the carotid tubercle, where the pulse of the common carotid artery in this area can be taken on this bone.

G) The transverse process of the seventh vertebra of the neck is completely covered by the clavicle and is not touched.

Spinous process of the cervical vertebrae (Spinuos process)

A) Spinous protrusion of the second cervical vertebra (C2): If you pull the fingertip down from the external protrusion (Inion) down in the midline, the first protrusion that may be touched will be the same protrusion, which is about 5-7 cm lower than The bulge will be posterior. If you bend your head, the midpoint of the distance between the inion and the spinal cord of the second vertebra (C2) indicates the large occipital fossa (Foramen magnum) from which to draw cerebrospinal fluid from a part of the subarachnoid space called the cerebellomedullary (Magna) cysterna. use.

B) The prickly appendages of the third to sixth vertebrae are covered by the occipital ligament (Nuchal ligament) and are not easily touched, and only in some people the prickly appendage of the sixth vertebra may be touched.

C) The thorny process of the seventh cervical vertebra is the most distinctive and palpable spinal process of the cervical vertebrae and is the first thorny process of the spine that can be easily touched from top to bottom in all people, even when standing, therefore as Vertebrae prominence Is called). This bulge is used as a marker to count the thoracic and lumbar vertebrae.

Chest vertebrae

Transverse zoom

They are long, thick and round, and gradually become smaller from beginning to end, but they are not palpable.

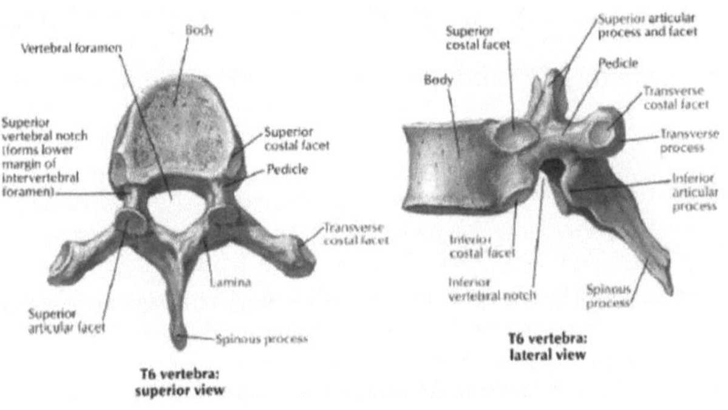

Figure 4. **Chest vertebrae**

The first and lower thoracic vertebrae have almost straight thorny appendages. The spinous appendages of the fourth to tenth vertebrae of the thorax are deflected downwards, and the apex of the vertebrae of a vertebra is flush with the lower vertebral body. Therefore, if it is necessary for the needle to enter the vertebral canal in these areas, the person should bend completely forward and insert the needle at an angle of 45 to 60 degrees. The thoracic vertebrae of the thorax are better characterized by bending forward. Counting vertebrae starts from the seventh vertebra of the neck down or from the level of the iliac crest (L4 and up). Or other anatomical signs of the back are used, such as the lower angle of the scapula. The spinous growths of the eleventh and twelfth thoracic vertebrae are straight and similar to the lumbar spine of the lumbar vertebrae.

A) The spinous process of the first thoracic vertebra (T1): is lower than the thorn of the seventh vertebra of the neck (C7) and more prominent than it.

B) Spinous process of the third thoracic vertebra (T3): It is almost flush with the inner end of the scapula and this mark can be used to count the rest of the thorns of the thoracic and lumbar vertebrae.

C) The spinous process of the seventh thoracic vertebra (T7): It is located approximately opposite the lower angle of the scapula.

D) The spinous process of the twelfth thoracic vertebra is located between the lower angle of the scapula (T7) and the highest point of the iliac crest (L4).

Lumbar vertebrae

Transverse process

The apex is about five centimeters to the midline and is covered by muscles.

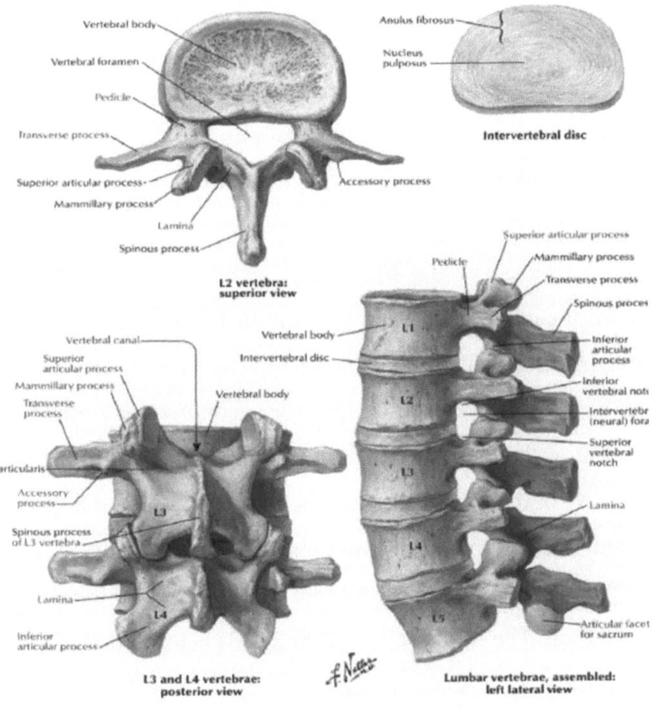

Figure 5. **Lumbar vertebrae**

Spinous process

The spines of the upper four lumbar vertebrae are recognizable separately. Especially if the person leans forward. If you connect the highest point of the iliac crest, the two sides pass through the fourth lumbar vertebra (L4). This is a very good sign for drawing cerebrospinal fluid (CSF) during lumbar puncture (LP). The space between the L4 and L5 blades is approximately 2.5 cm below this line (Supracristal line). The skin of this part is about 5 cm in adults and 2.5 cm in children to the space under the spider. The thorny appendages of the fifth lumbar vertebra are not easily touched.

Sacred beads

Median sacral crest

The spiny appendages of the upper sacral vertebrae fuse together to form the median sacral crest. The tip of the spines is palpable in adults as a spinous tubercle. The prickly growths of the fourth and fifth sacral vertebrae participate in the formation of the sacral hiatus.

A) The spinous process of the first sacral vertebra along with the fifth lumbar vertebra are located due to their location in the arch between the lumbar and sacral, they are not easily touched.

B) The spinous tubercle corresponding to the second sacral vertebra (S2) is located in the middle of the line connecting the posterior superior iliac spine (PSIS) on both sides. Also, the end of the subarachnoid space and the cerebrospinal fluid and the Anterior superior iliac spine (ASIS) are at this level, and the surface of the two PSIS passes through the middle of the sacroiliac joint.

C) Spinous tubercle The third sacral vertebra (S3) is located at the upper end of the natal cleft and is at the level of the upper right end of the rectum.

D) Sacral hiatus (Sacral hiatus) is located at the upper end of the neonatal cleft and 5 cm above the tail or 6 cm above the anus. If you move your fingers up from the tailbone, the hollow of the hiatus will become apparent in the lean person, and pressure in this area may cause pain. In some vertebral malformations, such as Spina bifida, the hiatus may be raised to a higher level. This lesion is sometimes so large that it causes a hernia of the spinal cord and meningeal membranes. Sometimes this defect is very weak and can only be detected on radiography.

Posterior sacral foramina

Sometimes it is necessary to find the location of the holes to anesthetize the sacral nerves separately. There are 4 sacral holes on each side. Follow the steps below to find the sacral holes. Cut the distance between the PSIS and the spinous tubercle in half and go up 3 cm from this point. The last point shows the location of the first sacral hole.

The second hole is 2.5 cm below the first hole or 0.5 cm above the midpoint between S2 and PSIS. The third hole is 2.5 cm away from the second hole. The fourth hole is 2.5 cm away from the third hole.

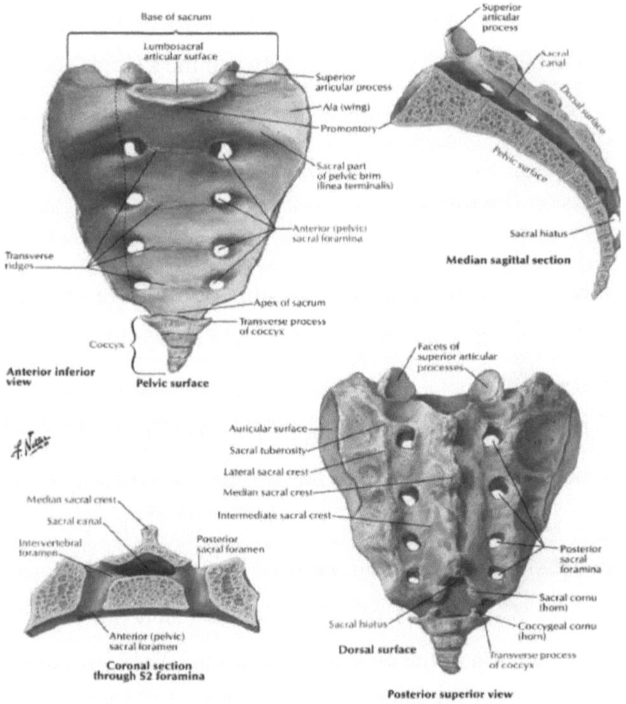

Figure 6. **Sacred beads**

Sacral promontary

The raised part of the upper edge of the body is called the first sacral vertebra. In lean people and at rest, sometimes you can put your fingers a few centimeters below the navel with a deep touch and gently but with increasing force put the abdomen in the middle line, you can hardly touch this bony protrusion. Sometimes you may confuse this bulge with a tumor. In women for examination, this bulge is used through the rectum and vagina to measure the diameter of the pelvis.

Tail bone

It is located deep in the congenital cleft and its lower end (apex) is about one centimeter above the anus. The anterior surface of this bone can be touched from inside the anus. The base of the bone is located above the congenital cleft and about 6 cm above the anus, which also shows the end of the sacral hiatus. Due to the fracture of the joints of different parts of the tail or the welded joint between the sacrum and the tail or the end of these joints, a very severe pain occurs. This condition is called Coccygodynia.

Other bony points on the back

Scapula

The palpable bony signs of the scapula in the upper limb were discussed, but here we re-examine the signs used to count the vertebrae and ribs or to find another building or place in the back.

The upper bouts featured two cutaways, for easier access to the higher frets. The inner end of the spine of the scapula is the surface of the spine of the third vertebra or the body of the fourth vertebra. In addition, the inner end of the scapula is on the fourth rib. This anatomical sign (scapula) can be used to count vertebrae or ribs. The inner side of the scapula is distinct and palpable, and just near its lower angle, this side participates in the formation of the ausculating triangle. The lower angle of the scapula is located at the level of the thorn of the seventh thoracic vertebra and on the seventh rib or the seventh space between the ribs, so the eighth rib is easily touched below it and can be used as a sign to count the ribs as well as the vertebrae.

Ribs

The ribs are easily touched a little further from the midline because near the vertebrae, the ribs are covered by the muscles of the erector spina. Sometimes it is impossible to touch the twelfth gear because it is short, and if the gear count starts from the bottom, the eleventh gear may be assumed to be the twelfth gear. This is especially important in kidney surgery. The kidney surgeon usually makes the incision below the 12th rib, and if the 12th rib is short, the surgeon makes the incision under the 11th rib, and the pleura and lung may rupture. To count the ribs on the back, two marks are used and the lower angle of the scapula is used (the inner end of the spine is on the fourth gear and the eighth gear is just below the lower angle). It belongs to the tenth rib, which is located on the sides and is level with the third lumbar vertebra and is about five centimeters away from the iliac crest.

Hip bone

Parts of this bone are touched in the back. The upper part of the iliac crest, which is level with the fourth lumbar vertebra, can be used as a marker for counting vertebrae or drawing cerebrospinal fluid (LP). PSIS In the skin dimple, about 4 cm of the midline is touched, which is equal to the level of the second sacral vertebra.

Lumbar puncture

Sometimes it is necessary to test for cerebrospinal fluid (CSF) or to inject anesthetic into the spinal cord or to use a radiograph to identify the ventricles of the brain. For all this, it is necessary for the needle to enter the subarachnoid space. The lower end of the spinal cord continues in the adult to the lower side of the first lumbar vertebra (L1) and in the infant to the third lumbar vertebra (L3). Therefore, the needle can be inserted into this space relatively safely. In this case, the vertebrae must be completely bent so that the space between the vertebrae is completely open.

For this purpose, the patient should be lying on one side or sitting. Needle into the space between the third and fourth vertebrae. (L3-L4) or the fourth and fifth lumbar (L4-L5) enter. To find the place to insert the needle, it is best to find the fourth lumbar vertebra. First find the highest point of the iliac crest and connect the right and left points with a transverse line and find the fourth vertebra of the lumbar vertebra and insert the needle at the top or bottom. The distance from the skin to the subarachnoid space is 5 cm in adults and 2.5 cm in children.

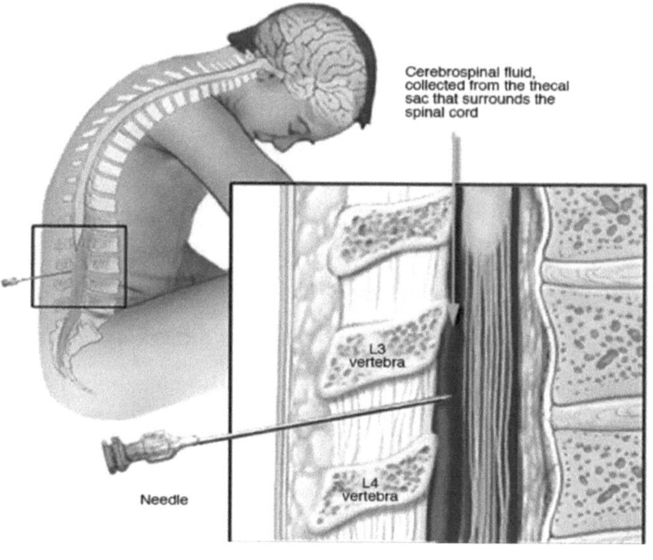

Figure 7. **Lumbar puncture**

Caudal or Spinal anesthesia

The anesthetic enters the extradural space through the sacral hiatus and numbs the spinal roots of the second, third, fourth, and fifth sacral nerves (S2-S5) and the coccygeal tail. This anesthesia is used in gynecological diseases to anesthetize the cervix and the perineum. To do this, insert the anesthetic at a 45 degree angle above the congenital cleft.

Muscles and back areas

There are four floors behind, some of which are palpable or visible.

Splenius capitis

It is a muscle that covers the floor of the back triangle of the neck and is characterized by resistance when straightening the neck.

Trapezius

It is a broad, triangular muscle with an upper angle at the external occipital protuberance, a lower angle at the dorsal spine (T12), and an external angle at the shoulders. By raising the shoulders against the resistance, the fibers of the upper part of the muscle are easily touched. More details about the next two muscles are given in the discussion of the upper limb.

Teres major

It is a thick muscle band located between the lower angle of the scapula and the humerus. This muscle, together with the latissimus dorsi, forms the dorsal fold of the axilla.

Latissimus dorsi

The lower outer edge of this muscle is along a line that extends from the middle of the iliac crest to the dorsal fold of the axilla, creating a bulge in this direction that becomes more pronounced during adduction to arm resistance.

Errector spina

It is located on both sides of the middle groove of the back and is well defined by its resistance to hyperextension. The work of these muscles is to control the spine and the curvature of the body position in the spine. To examine the muscles, both sides of the midline should be compared. If the muscles have a normal contraction, they are firm to the touch. Muscles that are in a state of muscle spasm are harder and shorter than muscles in the normal state, so that a convexity is seen on the vertebrae on the side where there is contraction.

Median posterior groove

It extends from the external occipital protuberance to the congenital cleft. Due to the irregularity of the back of the body, this groove has different depths in different areas, so that it is shallow in the neck area and is called Nuchal groove and is the deepest area in the upper back. This groove is in the form of a triangle in the lower part of the waist, the base of which is a linear triangle that connects the two PSIS, and its apex is at the upper end of the congenital cleft (S3).

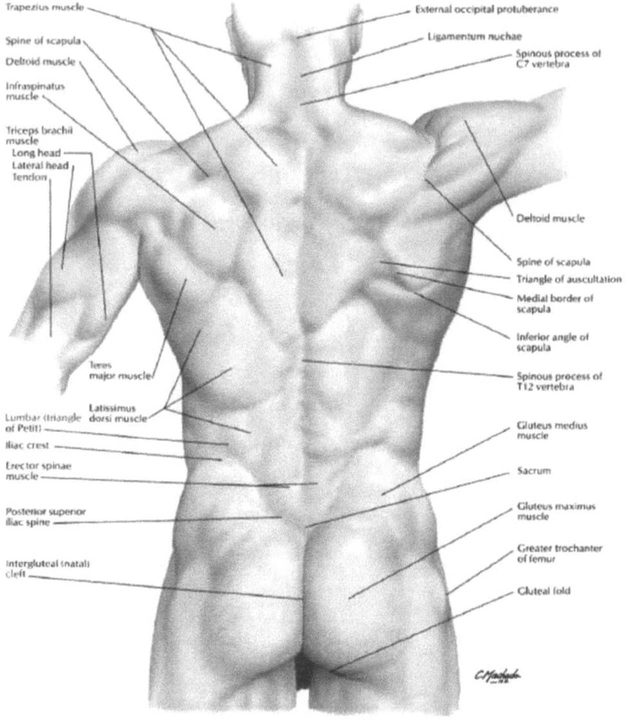

Figure 8. **Median posterior groove**

Skin dimple

There is a midline on the lower back on either side, each four inches from the centerline. PSIS can be touched below these depressions.

Natal cleft

It begins at the level of the third sacrum (S3) and extends to the anus.

Movements of the Back

The spiral appearance of the spine, which is composed of bony vertebrae and elastic intervertebral discs, has made this spine play a protective and protective role against impact. The movement between each of the two consecutive vertebrae is very small, but the sum of the total movements in the vertebral column is considerable and gives it considerable flexibility.

Movement is due to the partial flexibility of the intervertebral discs with the weakness of the synovial joint capsules located between the articular ridges. The semi-solid state of the disc nucleus (Nucleus pulposus) causes the pressure to be distributed evenly over the surface of the disc as the vertebrae move. The direction and amount of movements in different areas are mainly determined by the thickness of the intervertebral discs and the direction and shape of the joint appendages. Where the discs are thicker, the amount of movement increases. The neck is the most mobile part of the trunk and is responsible for moving the head towards the trunk. Trunk movements are more limited. The movements of the spine are as follows:

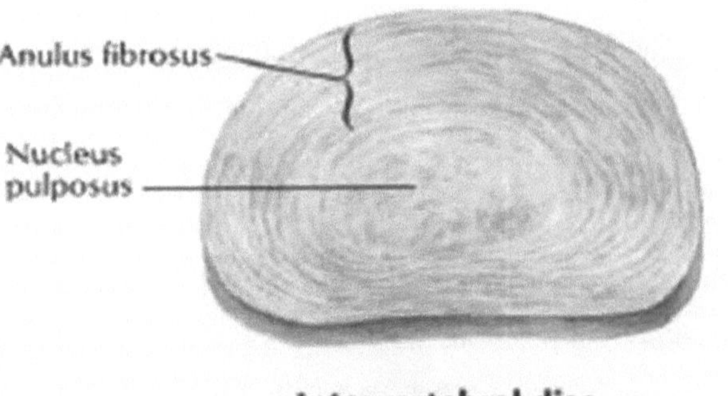

Figure 9. Intervertebral disc

Bending forward (Flexion)

In the neck area, where the discs are relatively thick, the movements are relatively extensive. In the upper parts of the chest, the intervertebral joints are located in such a way that they allow movement in a wide range, but due to the thin intervertebral discs, the presence of ribs and sternum and the stacking of the vertebrae bend forward. It is very limited. However, in the lower part of the chest, due to the greater flexibility of the cartilage and joints of the teeth and the presence of free ribs (ribs 11 and 12), the movements of this part are free. In the lumbar region, bending forward is largely possible, especially in the lumbar-sac joint (Lumbosacral), where the thickest intervertebral disc is located. If the forward bending movements are not well controlled, the discs may rupture. Abdominal mass is a barrier to bending forward, so it is easier to bend in lean people. When the abdominal mass bends, it pushes the diaphragm upwards and reduces the ability to breathe.

When bending forward, such as touching the toes, most movements occur in the pelvic joints, and the lumbar vertebrae move less. The main forward movement of the spine is mainly due to the flexion of the pelvic joint and the joints between the atlas and the occipital joint (Atlanto-occipital joint). When bending forward, the lumbar curvature decreases.

Leaning back (Extension)

The amount of straightening of the spine is more than the amount of forward bending of the spine. There is the greatest amount of straightening (Extension) in the neck and waist areas. In the neck area, it is possible to bend backwards. In the lumbar region, some straightening occurs, especially in the lumbar joint to the sacrum where the disc is thick. At extension, the freest area is the lower back (L4-L5). For example, if a heavy object is lifted in an upright position, the possibility of injury to this area is very high, unless good muscle control is exercised, especially by the abdominal muscles.

Lateral flexion

In the neck area, articular surfaces cause bending to the sides and rotation to occur together. Therefore, it bends to one side with a slight rotation to the other side. Bending to the sides occurs mainly in the lumbar and thoracic regions. The range of motion varies from person to person and depends on the shape of the body. The closer the gearbox is to the Iliac crest, the greater the restriction of movement, so in thin and tall people this movement is easier than in short and wide people.

Rotation

Spinal rotation can occur in the neck and chest area. Articular lumbar vertebrae prevent any rotation in the lumbar region. In the thoracic region, although rotation is theoretically possible, this rotation is limited by the thorax. The sternum acts as a splint for the upper half of the chest. Therefore, the rotation can be done only in the lower half and there is a maximum rotation in the area of free gears (gears 11 and 12). When the chest rotates left and right. Because there is no rotation in the upper chest and waist, an S-shaped curvature is revealed in the lower chest. Although proper control of each vertebra is provided by the small intervertebral muscles, the main efficiency of trunk rotation is provided by the internal oblique muscles (Obliqus internus abdominis) and the external abdominal muscles (Obliqus externus abdominus). The internal oblique muscle of one side works together with the external oblique muscle of the opposite side.

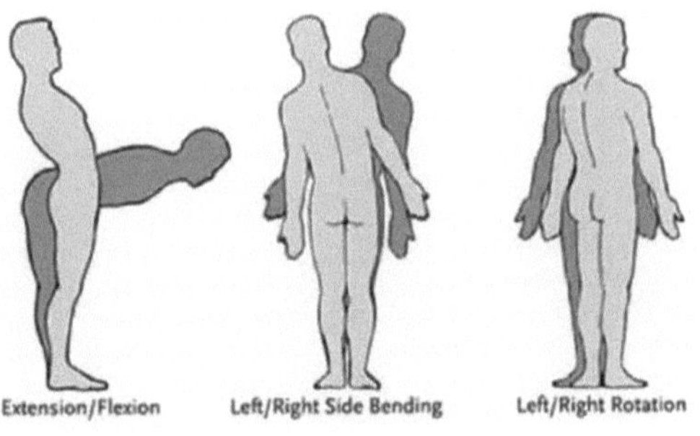

Figure 10. Rotation

Back pain

Minor back pain is very common but only a small percentage of the material is due to disc herniation. This type of pain may be caused by a sudden movement of the spine, especially a forward bending motion. In general, the most common cause of low back pain, which is mostly in the lower back (Low back pain) are:

1) Intervertebral disc herniation
2) vertebral fractures
3) Inflammation of the synovial joints between the vertebrae (Arthritis)
4) Rupture or stretching of the intervertebral ligaments
5) Spasm of the back muscles
6) Spinal curvature abnormalities.

Chapter II

Gastrointestinal Tract

Mouth

The mouth has 2 parts:

- ✓ Atrium: The space between the teeth and lips (in front) and the cheeks (on the sides).
- ✓ The main cavity of the mouth: It is filled with the tongue.

The mucosa of each lip has a crease in the middle line called the Frenulum of the lip that connects the lip to the mucosa on the inner surface of the lip.

Palate: The roof of the mouth or the floor of the nasal cavity. It has 2 sections:

- ✓ Hard palate: It forms two anterior thirds of the palate and is composed of maxillary and palatine bones.
- ✓ Soft palate: It forms the posterior third of the palate and contains fibrous tissue and muscles in its thickness.

The soft palate muscles are:

- ✓ Tensor veli palatine.
- ✓ Soft palate muscle (Levator veli palatine).
- ✓ Palatoglossus muscle.
- ✓ Palatopharyngeal muscle.
- ✓ Small tongue muscle (Uvula).

Tooth

- ✓ The number of deciduous teeth is 20 and the number of permanent teeth is 32.

Number of teeth in each hemisphere:

- ✓ front teeth (Incisors).
- ✓ Fang (Canine).
- ✓ teeth of Asia Minor (Premolar).
- ✓ teeth of Greater Asia (Molar).

The teeth of Asia Minor do not have deciduous teeth.

Each tooth consists of 3 parts:

- ✓ Crown: The part that is visible.
- ✓ Neck: The part between the crown and the root that is covered by the gums.
- ✓ Root: The part of the tooth that is located inside the jaw bones.

In the incision made from the thickness of the tooth, there are the following areas:
- ✓ Enamel.
- ✓ Dentin (Dentine).
- ✓ Cement.
- ✓ Periodontium ligaments.

Tongue

The villi of the tongue are:
- ✓ Filiform villi: No taste buds.
- ✓ Fungal villi (Fungiform).
- ✓ Jaw or valley (Circumvallate).
- ✓ Foliate.

Between the anterior two-thirds and the posterior one-third of the dorsal surface of the tongue is the terminal sulcus (Sulcus terminalis).

The lingual tonsils are located in the posterior third of the dorsal surface of the tongue.

The lower surface of the tongue is attached to the floor mucosa by the Frenulum of the tongue.

For information on tongue muscles, refer to the muscle chapter.

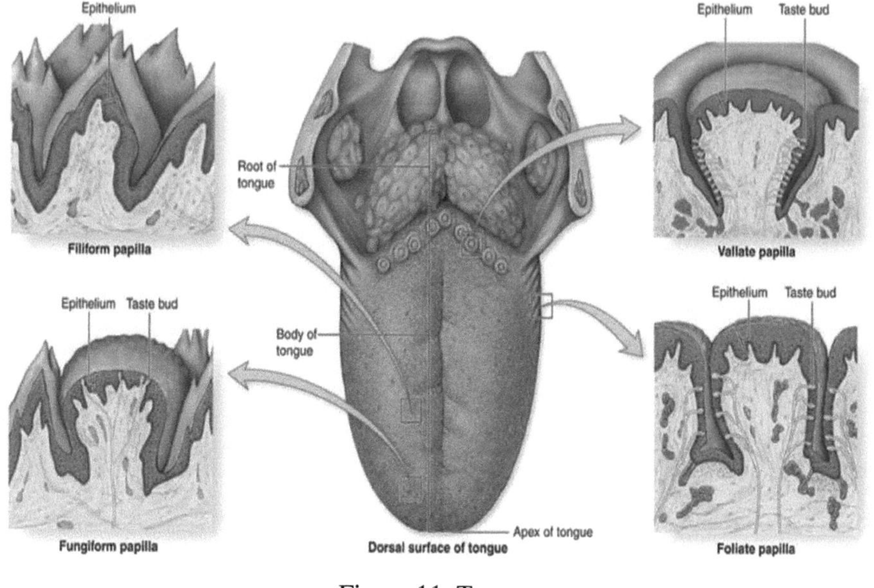

Figure 11. Tongue

Lines and areas of the abdomen

In one of the anatomical divisions, the abdomen can be divided into 9 areas by 4 lines.

These four lines are:

- ✓ 2 midclavicular lines: Pass through the middle of the clavicle.
- ✓ Transpyloric line: Passes through the pyloric valve.
- ✓ Intertecular line: Passes through the right and left buttons.

The nine areas of the abdomen are:

- ✓ 1 epigastric region.
- ✓ 1 Hypogastric region.
- ✓ 2 lumbar regions (lumbar).
- ✓ 1 navel area.
- ✓ 2 hypochondriac regions.
- ✓ 2 inguinal area.

Peritoneum

The peritoneum has two parts, both of which are parallel to each other:
- ✓ Peritoneal wall: covers the inner surface of the abdominal wall.
- ✓ Visceral peritoneum: Located on the viscera.

The space between these two layers is called the peritoneal cavity. The peritoneal cavity is a closed cavity in men, but in women it communicates with the outside environment through the vagina, uterus, and fallopian tubes.

Abdominal viscera can be divided into 2 categories based on peritoneal lining:
- ✓ Intraperitoneal viscera: All surfaces of this viscera (anterior, posterior, and lateral surfaces) are completely covered by the peritoneum. The visceral peritoneum, after completely covering the viscera, forms a two-layered membrane called the meso; Arteries and nerves pass through the thickness of the meso and enter the viscera.

Intraperitoneal viscera are:
- ✓ Stomach (except bare area).
- ✓ 2.5 cm from the beginning of the duodenum.
- ✓ Ileum;
- ✓ Appendix;
- ✓ Cecum (inside the peritoneum, but lacks meso);
- ✓ Colon transverse;
- ✓ Colon sigmoid;
- ✓ Liver (except bare area);
- ✓ Pancreas tail;
- ✓ The spleen;
- ✓ Rahm;

Extraperitoneal viscera: These are viscera whose peritoneum covers only part of the surface (not completely) and are attached directly to the posterior wall of the abdomen.

Extraperitoneal viscera are:

- ✓ Abdominal esophagus;
- ✓ Duodenum (except for the first 2.5 cm);
- ✓ Bare area of the stomach;
- ✓ Ascending colon;
- ✓ Descending colon;
- ✓ Kidneys;
- ✓ Adrenal glands.
- ✓ Ureters.
- ✓ Pancreas (except tail).
- ✓ Naked area of the liver.
- ✓ Aorta.
- ✓ Lower Wisconsin.
- ✓ Bladder.
- ✓ Rectum.

Note

- ✓ The presence of meso causes visceral motility; The longer the meso, the greater the mobility of the limb.
- ✓ The extraperitoneal viscera are not motile due to lack of meso.

The peritoneal cavity has two parts, which are connected by a Winslow hole or an omental hole (Omental or Winslow foreman):

- ✓ Lesser sac: The space at the back of the stomach.
- ✓ Er Greater sac

Important peritoneal derivatives are:

- ✓ Er Greater omentum: Attached to the large curvature of the stomach.

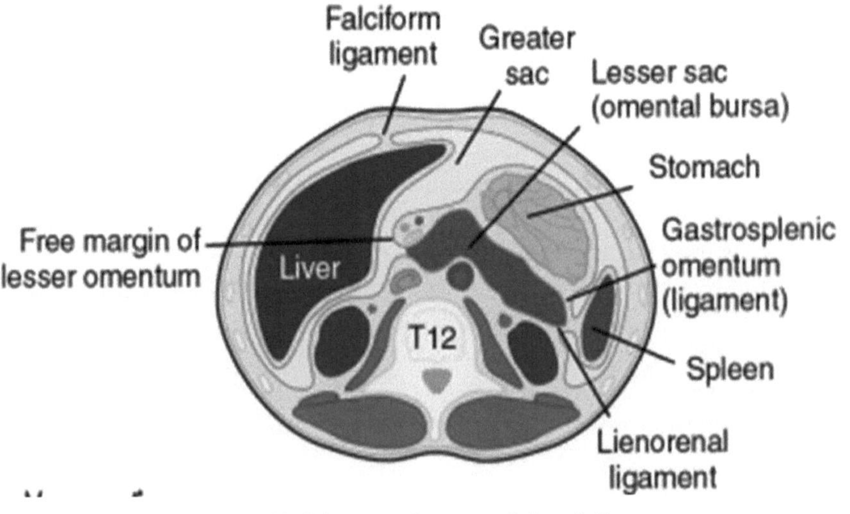

Figure 12. Lines and areas of the abdomen

✓ Lesser omentum: The small curvature of the stomach and the initial part of the duodenum connects to the liver.

✓ Falciform ligament: Attaches the anterior surface of the liver to the posterior surface of the abdominal wall.

✓ Round hepatic ligament: Attaches the lower free side of the liver to the umbilicus.

✓ Right and left coronary ligaments of the liver: Attaches the upper surface of the liver to the diaphragm.

✓ Gastrosplenic ligament: Attaches the stomach to the spleen.

✓ Splenural ligament: Attaches the spleen to the left kidney.

✓ Gastrocolic ligament: Attaches the stomach to the large intestine.

✓ Broad ligament.

✓ Ovarian hanging ligament.

Important peritoneal implants:

✓ Rectovesical pouch.

- ✓ Rectouterine pouch.
- ✓ Uterovesical pouch.

Esophagus

- ✓ Its length is 25 cm.
- ✓ It extends from the throat (in the C6 vertebrae) to the stomach.

It has 3 sections:

- ✓ Neck section.
- ✓ Chest section.
- ✓ Abdominal part.

There are 4 strictures along the esophagus, which are:

- ✓ The first stenosis: at the junction of the throat.
- ✓ Second stenosis: adjacent to the aortic arch.
- ✓ Third stenosis: adjacent to the left main bronchus.
- ✓ Fourth stenosis: where it passes through the diaphragm hole.

Adjacent to the esophagus:

- ✓ Anterior (top to bottom): trachea, pericardium and diaphragm.
- ✓ Posterior: The trunk of the thoracic vertebrae and the descending aorta.
- ✓ On the right: the right lung and its associated pleura.
- ✓ Left: Left lung and associated pleura, aortic arch and descending aorta.

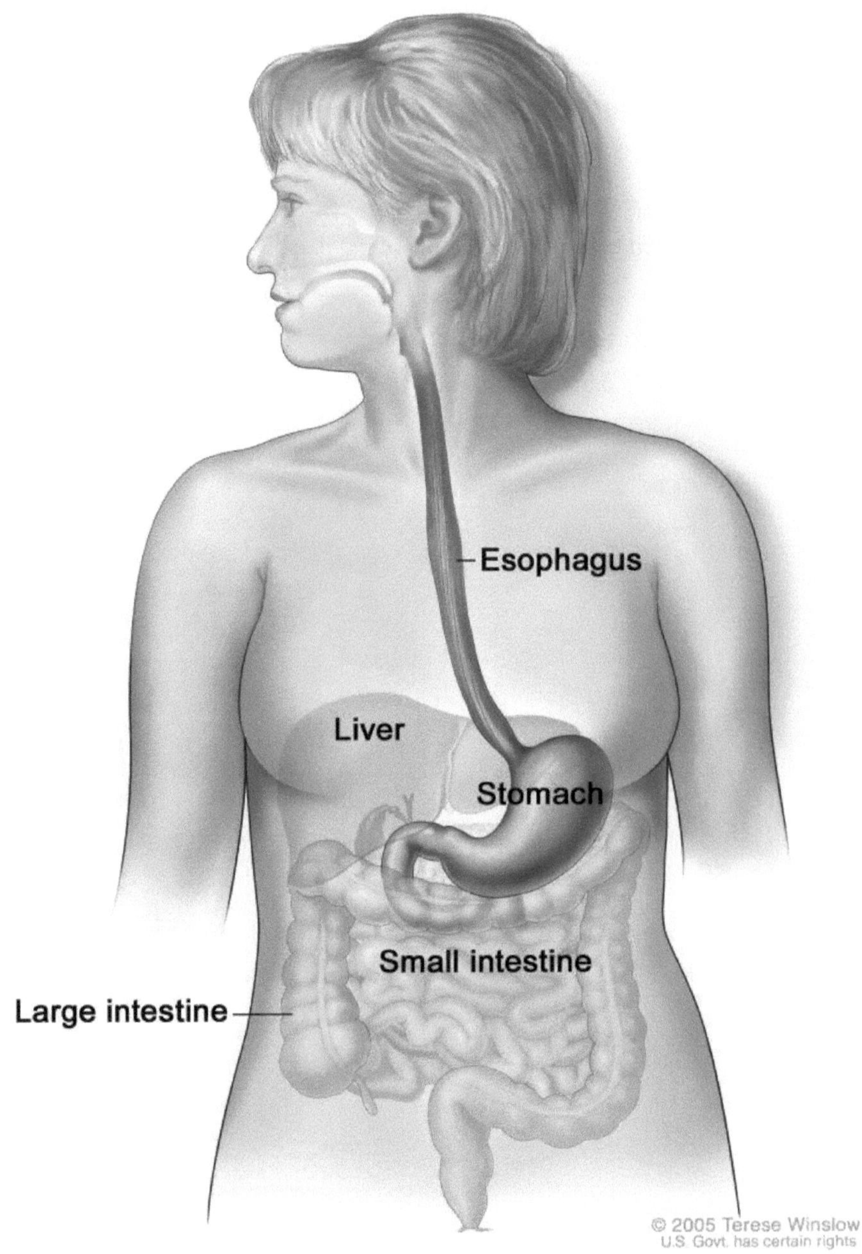

Figure 13. Esophagus

✓

Stomach

The stomach has 4 parts:

- ✓ Cardia: The esophagus attaches to it.
- ✓ Fundus: It is located below the left dome of the diaphragm and usually contains air.
- ✓ Body: The largest part of the stomach.
- ✓ Pyloric part: (Pyloric part): It has 2 parts:
- ✓ Antrum.
- ✓ Pilor Channel.

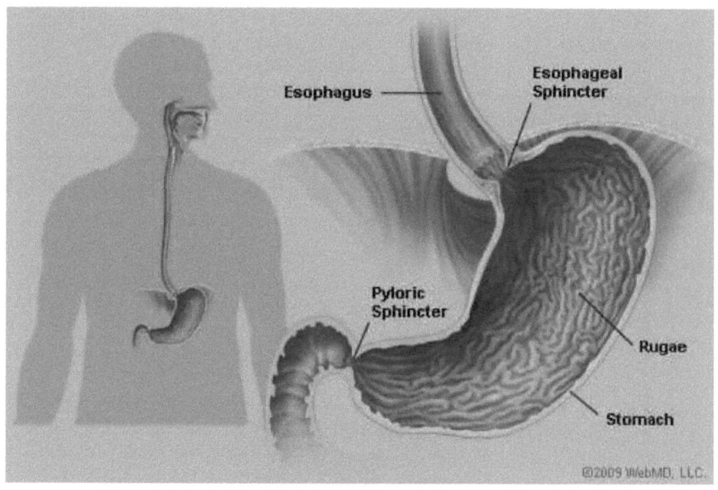

Figure 14. Stomach

- ✓ The angle between the esophagus and the gastric fundus is called the cardiac notch.
- ✓ At the end of the pyloric canal, the thickness of the annular muscles of the stomach wall increases and forms the pyloric sphincter. The pyloric sphincter is located around the L1 vertebra and to the right of the midline of the abdomen.
- ✓ The longitudinal folds of the inner surface of the stomach are called Ruger.

The stomach has 2 curvatures:

- ✓ Small curvature: Angular notch is located in this curvature. This incision defines the boundary between the trunk and the pyloric region. The small curvature of the stomach is attached to the small tentacle.
- ✓ Large curvature: A large tent is attached to it.

Adjacent to the stomach:

- ✓ Anterior: diaphragm, left lobe of liver, anterior abdominal wall
- ✓ Posterior: Diaphragm, spleen, left kidney, left adrenal gland, pancreas and transverse colon
- ✓ Stomach arteries and nerves:
- ✓ Arteries: celiac trunk branches
- ✓ Veins: Drain directly and indirectly into the portal vein.
- ✓ Lymph: Discharged to celiac nodes.
- ✓ Nerves: includes sympathetic and parasympathetic and is supplied by the celiac neural network.

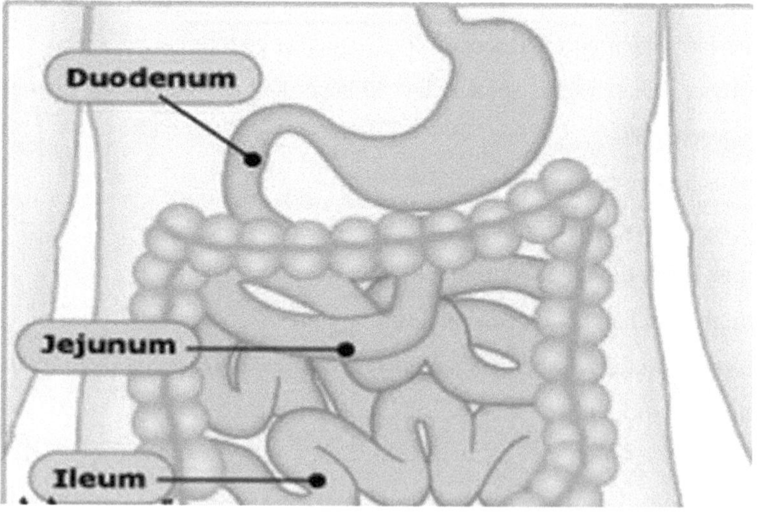

Figure 15. Artry in stomach

Small intestine

The small intestine has 3 parts:

- ✓ Duodenum or duodenum

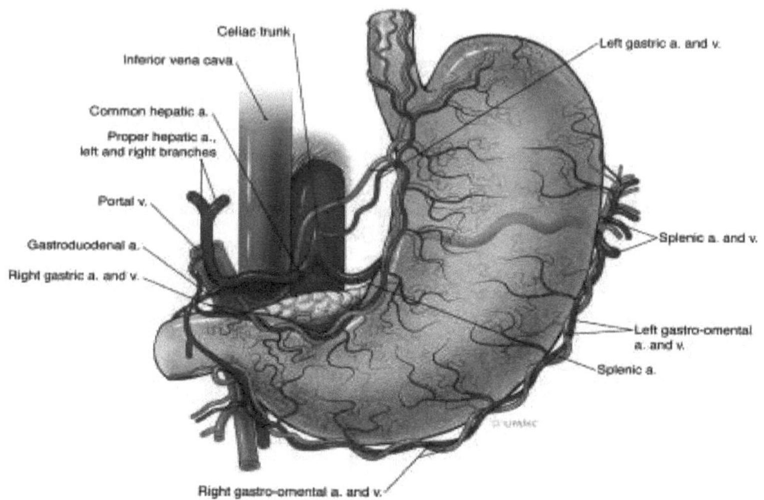

Figure 16. Adjacent to the stomach

✓ It is 25 cm long.

✓ It is C-shaped and surrounds the head of the pancreas.

✓ The beginning ends at the pylorus and the end at the duodenum bend.

The duodenum has 4 sections:

✓ The first part (upper part): is 5 cm and in front and on the right side is the body of L1 nut.

✓ The second part (descending part): is 8 cm. To the right is the L1 - L3 nut. Inside the duct of the second part of the duodenum, two protrusions are visible:

1) Major duodenal papilla: The main duct of the pancreas and the common bile duct are emptied at this point.

2) Minor duodenal papilla: The pancreatic duct (Santorini duct) enters it.

✓ Third part (horizontal part): 7 cm. Located at the level of the L3 vertebra. It passes through the front of the aorta and the inferior vena cava.

✓ The fourth part (ascending part): 5 cm. To the left are the L2 and L3 beads.

Note

✓ The junction of the duodenum with the jejunum is called the duodenojejunal flexure. This bend is connected to the right column of the diaphragm by the treitz ligament or Suspensory muscle of the duodenum.

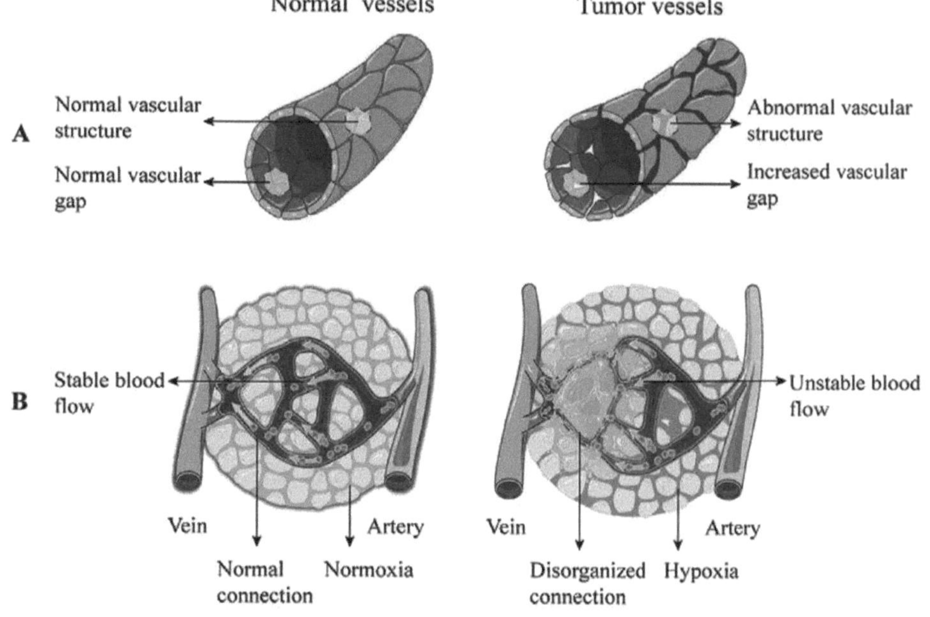

Figure 17. Differences between ileal and geogenic tissues

Duodenal arteries and nerves

- ✓ Arteries: celiac trunk branches and upper mesenteric arteries.
- ✓ Veins: Drain into the port system.
- ✓ Lymph: Discharges to the celiac nodes and the upper mesenteric nodes.
- ✓ Nerves: It consists of sympathetic and parasympathetic and is supplied by the celiac neural network and the upper mesenteric network.

Jejunum and ileum

- ✓ The jejunum is mostly in the upper left quadrant of the abdomen.
- ✓ The ileum is mostly located in the lower right quadrant of the abdomen.
- ✓ The jejunum and ileum are attached to the posterior wall of the abdomen by the mesentery.

Some of the anatomical differences between the jejunum and the ileum are:
- ✓ The wall thickness and diameter of the jejunum lumen are larger than the ileum.
- ✓ The annular mucosal folds in the jejunum are larger and larger.
- ✓ In the lining of the ileum, accumulations of lymph nodes called Peyer's patches are visible.

The arteries and nerves of the jejunum and ileum
- ✓ Artery: Upper mesenteric artery
- ✓ Veins: It flows into the portal vein through the upper mesenteric vein.
- ✓ Lymph: It drains into the upper mesenteric lymph nodes.
- ✓ Nerves: includes sympathetic and parasympathetic and is supplied by the upper mesenteric neural network.

Colon

General features of the large intestine:
- ✓ It has a larger diameter than the small intestine.
- ✓ It has a piece-by-piece view and bags called Haustra.
- ✓ The longitudinal muscles accumulate in the wall of the colon and form 3 Teniae coli.
- ✓ At the level of the colon, peritoneal appendages containing fat called omental appendices are visible.

The large intestine has 8 parts:
- ✓ Cecum
- ✓ Appendix
- ✓ Ascending colon
- ✓ Transverse colon
- ✓ Descending colon
- ✓ Sigmoid colon
- ✓ Rectum

✓ Anal canal

Blind or cecal intestine

✓ The first part is the large intestine.

✓ The end of the ileum and appendix are connected to it.

✓ The junction of the ileum and vasculitis is called the ileocecal junction, where there is a valve of the same name. This valve has 2 anterior and posterior frenulum.

✓ The cecum is located in the right iliac cavity.

✓ It is supplied by branches of the upper mesenteric artery.

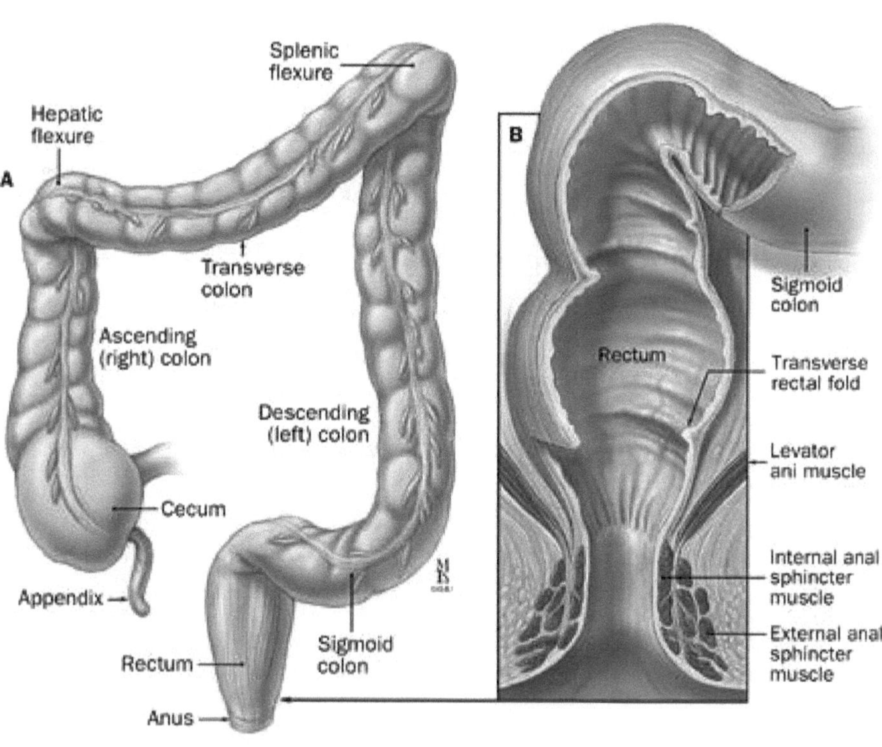

Figure 18. cecal intestine

Appendix

- ✓ The appendage is about 10-6 cm protruding from the posterior-inner wall of the cecum.
- ✓ The appendix has a meso called the mesoappendix.

Appendix arteries and nerves:

- ✓ Artery: A branch of the upper mesenteric artery supplies blood through the appendicular artery.
- ✓ Lymph: Discharges to the upper mesenteric nodes.
- ✓ Nerves: includes sympathetic and parasympathetic and is supplied by the upper mesenteric neural network.

Ascending colon

- ✓ On the right side, the abdomen extends from the cecum to below the liver.
- ✓ It is supplied by branches of the upper mesenteric artery.

Note

- ✓ The border between the ascending colon and the transverse colon is called the right colic flexion or hepatic flexion (due to its proximity to the liver).
- ✓ The border between the transverse colon and the descending colon is called the right colic flexion or splenic flexion. (Due to proximity to the spleen).
- ✓ The left colic flexion is higher than the right colic flexion.

Colon transverse

- ✓ The largest part is the large intestine.
- ✓ It has a meso called the transverse mesocolon.
- ✓ It extends from the right colic flexion to the left colic flexion.

Transverse colon vessels and nerves

- ✓ Artery: It is supplied by branches of the upper mesenteric and inferior mesenteric arteries.
- ✓ Lymph: It drains into the upper mesenteric and inferior mesenteric lymph nodes.
- ✓ Nerves: It consists of sympathetic and parasympathetic and is supplied by the upper mesenteric and inferior mesenteric neural networks.
- ✓

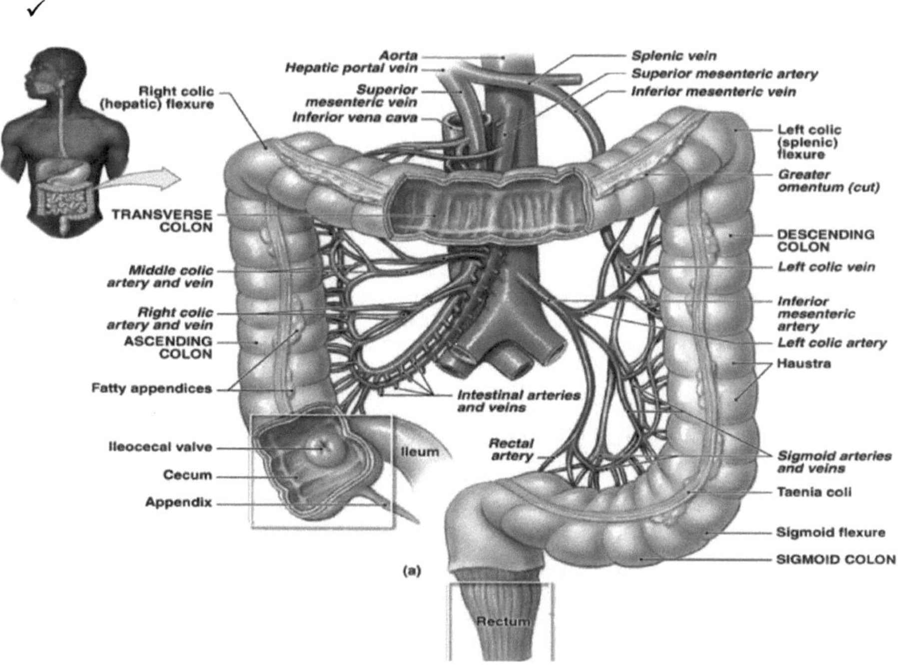

Figure 19. Transverse colon vessels and nerves

Descending colon
- ✓ On the left side of the abdomen is stretched from the left colic to the sigmoid.

Descending Colon Arteries and Nerves:
- ✓ Artery: It is bloodied by branches of the inferior mesenteric artery.
- ✓ Lymph: Discharges to the lower mesenteric nodes.
- ✓ Nerves: It includes the sympathetic and parasympathetic nerves and is supplied by the inferior mesenteric neural network.

Colon sigmoid
- ✓ It is S-shaped and extends from the end of the descending colon to the front of the S3 vertebra and eventually connects to the rectum. The junction of the sigmoid with the rectum is called the rectosigmoid junction.
- ✓ The origin of its arteries and nerves is similar to that of the descending colon.

Rectum or rectum
- ✓ It extends from the rectosigmoid junction to the anal canal. The junction of the rectum with the anal canal is called the anorectal junction.
- ✓ It lacks tapeworm.
- ✓ It has 3 lateral curves (upper, middle and lower). The upper and lower curves are on the right and the middle curve is on the left.
- ✓ It has a posterior anterior curvature called the sacral curvature.
- ✓ Its mucosa has 3 annular folds (upper, middle and lower). The upper and lower folds are on the left and the middle fold is on the right.
- ✓ The rectum is enlarged in a part of itself called the ampulla.

Adjacent to the rectum:
- ✓ Anteriorly: In men, it is adjacent to the base of the bladder, ureters, seminal vesicles, vas deferens, and prostate. In women, it is adjacent to the vagina.

✓ Posterior: S3 - S5 vertebrae and tailbone.

Rectal arteries and nerves

✓ Artery: It is supplied by branches of the inferior mesenteric artery and the internal iliac artery.

✓ Vein: There is ortho-venous communication in the rectal wall.

✓ Lymph: It drains into the inferior mesenteric lymph nodes and the internal iliac.

✓ Nerves: includes the sympathetic and parasympathetic and is supplied by the hypogastric networks of the pelvis.

Anal canal

✓ It is the end of the colon and extends from the anorectal junction to the anus.

✓ The upper part of the anal canal is covered with mucus and the lower part is covered with skin.

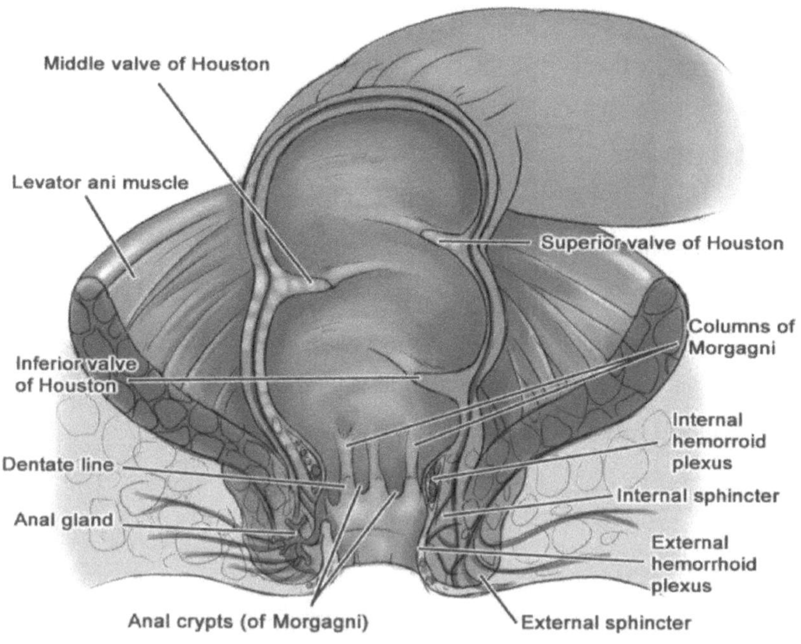

Figure 20. Anal canal

There are two types of sphincters around the anus:
- ✓ Internal sphincter: It is composed of annular smooth muscle and is involuntary.
- ✓ External sphincter: It is composed of skeletal muscle and is voluntary.

In the mucosa of the canal, there are anal columns, the lower edge of which are called anal valves. Above each of the valves is a space called the anal sinuses.
The lower limit of the valves forms an irregular line called the pectinate line.
1 cm below the shoulder line is the border between the skin and the mucosa, which is called the skin-anal line (Anocutaneuous line).

Anal canals and nerves
- ✓ Artery: It is supplied by branches of the internal iliac artery.
- ✓ Lymph: Discharges to the internal iliac and superficial inguinal nodes.
- ✓ Nerves: include sympathetic and parasympathetic (from the lower hypogastric networks) and somatic nerves (from the sacral nerves).

Pancreas

In appearance, the pancreas has four parts:
- ✓ Head: Surrounded by the duodenum. An appendage of it is called the inward process (Uncinate process).
- ✓ Neck
- ✓ Trunk: It has 3 upper, lower and anterior sides, to which the anterior root of the transverse mesoculon is connected.
- ✓ Tail: Located in the thickness of the splenorenal ligament.

In the thickness of the pancreas, there are 2 ducts:
- ✓ Main duct or Virsung: Its end connects to the common bile duct and drains into the second part of the duodenum. The accumulation of annular muscles around where they enter the duodenum is called the Oddi sphincter.

✓ Duct or Santorini: The end of it drains separately into the second part of the duodenum.

Pancreatic arteries and nerves

✓ Arteries: Branches of the celiac trunk and upper mesenteric artery

✓ Veins: Venous blood is drained to the portal vein through the spleen and upper mesenteric veins.

✓ Lymph: Discharged to the upper celiac and mesenteric nodes.

✓ Nerves: includes sympathetic and parasympathetic and is supplied by the celiac and mesenteric neural networks.

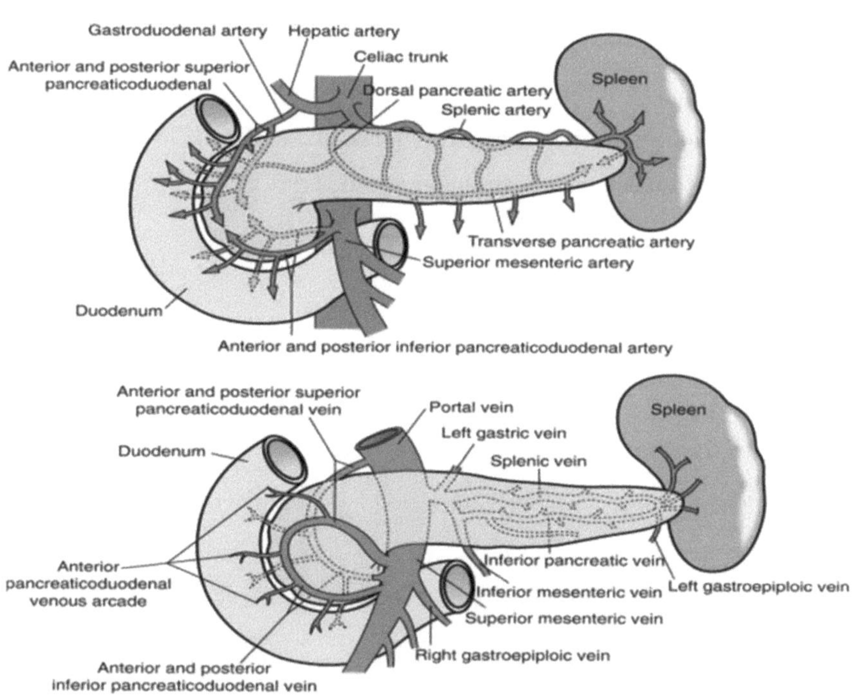

Figure 21. Pancreas

Liver

The liver is located in the following abdominal areas:

- ✓ Right hypochondriac region.
- ✓ Epigastric region.
- ✓ Left hypochondriac region.

Anatomically, the liver has 4 lobes:

- ✓ Right lobe.
- ✓ Left lobe.
- ✓ Caudate.
- ✓ Quadrate.

It has 2 levels:

- ✓ Diaphragmatic surface: Falciform ligament separating the right and left lobes in the anterior part.
- ✓ Visceral level: The following can be seen in the visceral surface of the liver:

1) Porta hepatis: The portal vein, hepatic artery and common bile duct pass through it.
2) Visceral effects: gallbladder, stomach, duodenum, colon, kidney and right adrenal gland.
3) Lower Wisconsin.
4) Round ligament.
5) Venous ligament (Ligamentum venosum).

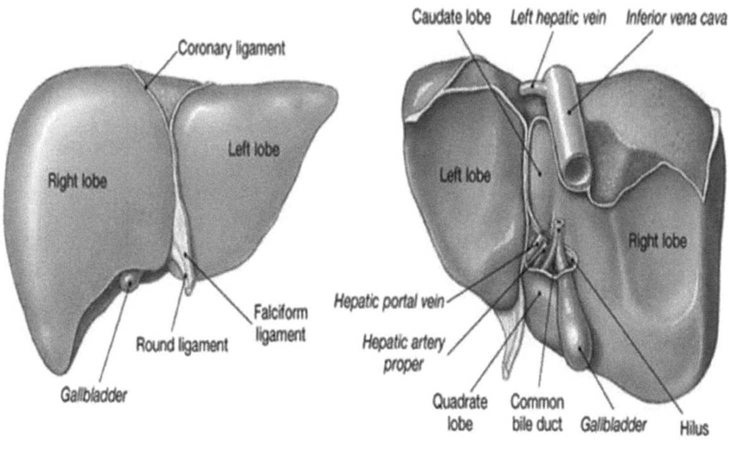

Figure 22. Liver

Square Lobe Range:

- ✓ Upper limit: umbilical cord
- ✓ Right: Gallbladder
- ✓ Left border: round hepatic ligament
- ✓ Lower limit: The lower edge of the liver

Lips of the tail:

- ✓ Lower limit: umbilical cord
- ✓ Right: Lower Wisconsin
- ✓ Left border: venous ligament

The liver has 8 segments, each of which has a separate blood supply and bile duct.

Hepatic arteries and nerves

- ✓ Artery: Hepatic artery (a branch of the celiac trunk).
- ✓ Vein: Port.
- ✓ Hepatic veins: Drain into the lower vena cava. These veins are one of the factors that keep the liver in place.
- ✓ Lymph: Discharged to celiac nodes.
- ✓ Nerves: includes sympathetic and parasympathetic and is supplied by the celiac network.

Bile ducts

✓ The path of bile from the moment it is made in the liver to enter the gallbladder:

✓ The bile duct from the gallbladder to the second part.

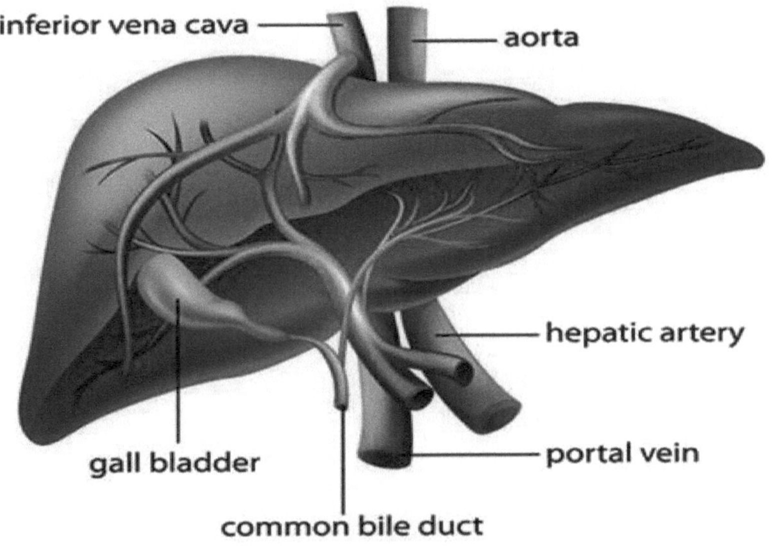

Figure 23. Bile ducts

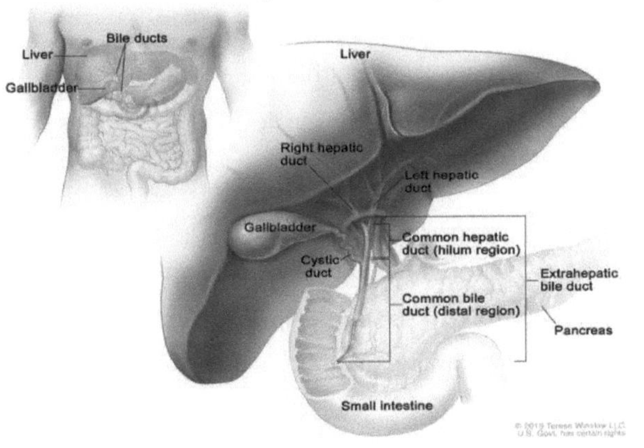

Figure 24. Bile ducts

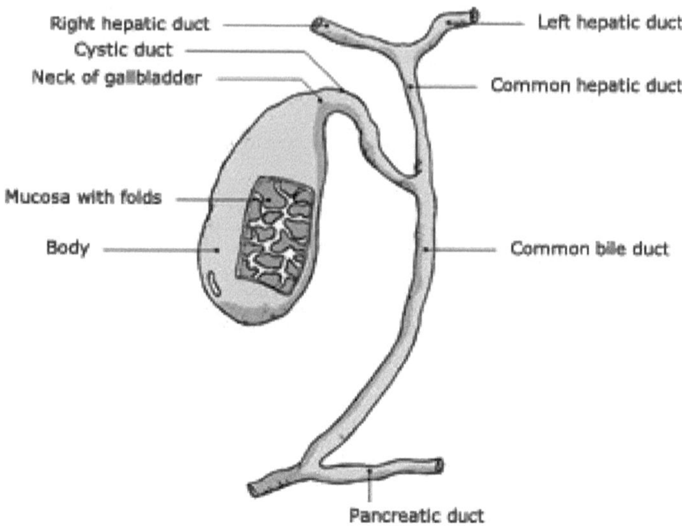

Figure 25. gallbladder

Duodenum

Gallbladder (Galblader)

The gallbladder has the following parts:

- ✓ Fundus: The widest part of the gallbladder and protrudes from the lower edge of the liver.
- ✓ Body.
- ✓ Neck: The narrowest part of the gallbladder. It has a spiral valve called a spiral valve. The neck is located along the cystic duct.

Gallbladder vessels and nerves

- ✓ Cystic artery: A branch of the common hepatic artery.
- ✓ Its venous blood drains into the port vein.
- ✓ Lymph: Drain into the celiac lymph nodes.
- ✓ Nerves: includes sympathetic and parasympathetic and is supplied by the celiac network.

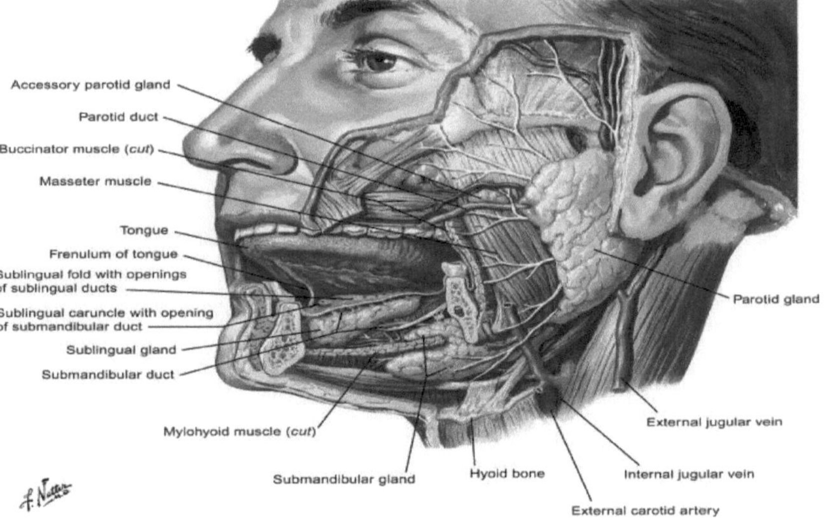

Figure 26. Gallbladder vessels and nerves

Salivary glands

- ✓ Parotid gland.
- ✓ Submandibular gland.
- ✓ Sublingual gland.

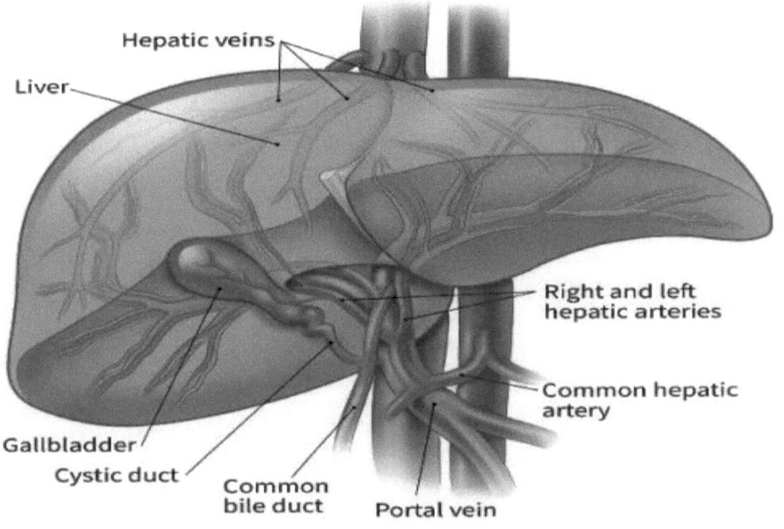

Figure 27. Salivary glands

Parotid gland

- ✓ It is located in front of the ear
- ✓ Its canal opens to the inner surface of the cheek adjacent to the second tooth of the Greater Asia Minor.
- ✓ Its blood supply is responsible for the external carotid artery.
- ✓ Its innervation is provided by the auriculotemporal nerve (a branch of the mandibular nerve).

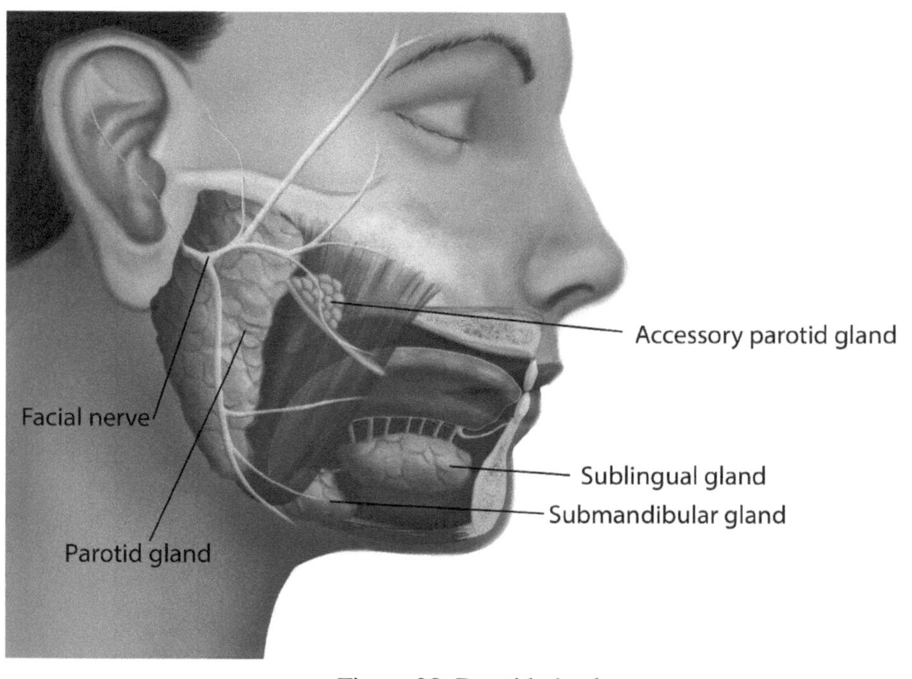

Figure 28. Parotid gland

Submandibular gland

This gland has 2 parts:

- ✓ Superficial: Located below the myeloid muscle. This part is palpable on the lower side of the mandibular bone.
- ✓ Deep section: Located above the myeloid muscle.

The secretions of this gland are discharged through the corresponding duct to the papilla in the floor of the mouth.

Its blood supply is provided through the facial (pink) artery.

The lingual nerve (a branch of the mandibular nerve) innervates it.

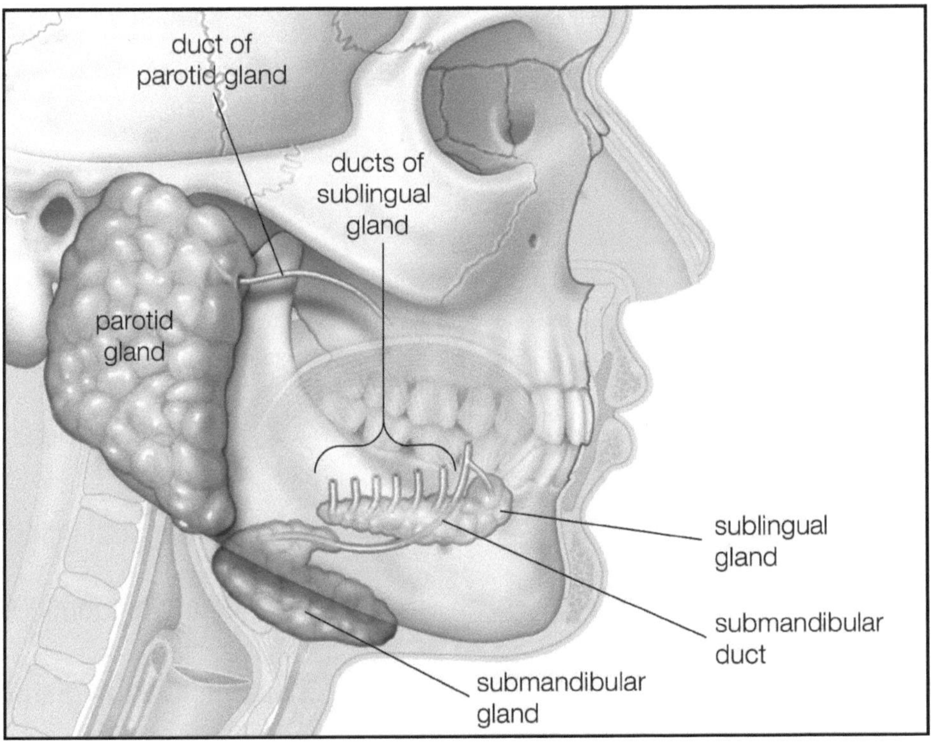

Figure 29. Submandibular gland

Sublingual gland

- ✓ It is located at the top of the myeloid muscle.
- ✓ Its secretions are discharged to the edge of the sublingual crease of the floor of the mouth.
- ✓ Its blood supply is provided through the facial (pink) and lingual arteries.
- ✓ The lingual nerve (a branch of the mandibular nerve) innervates it.

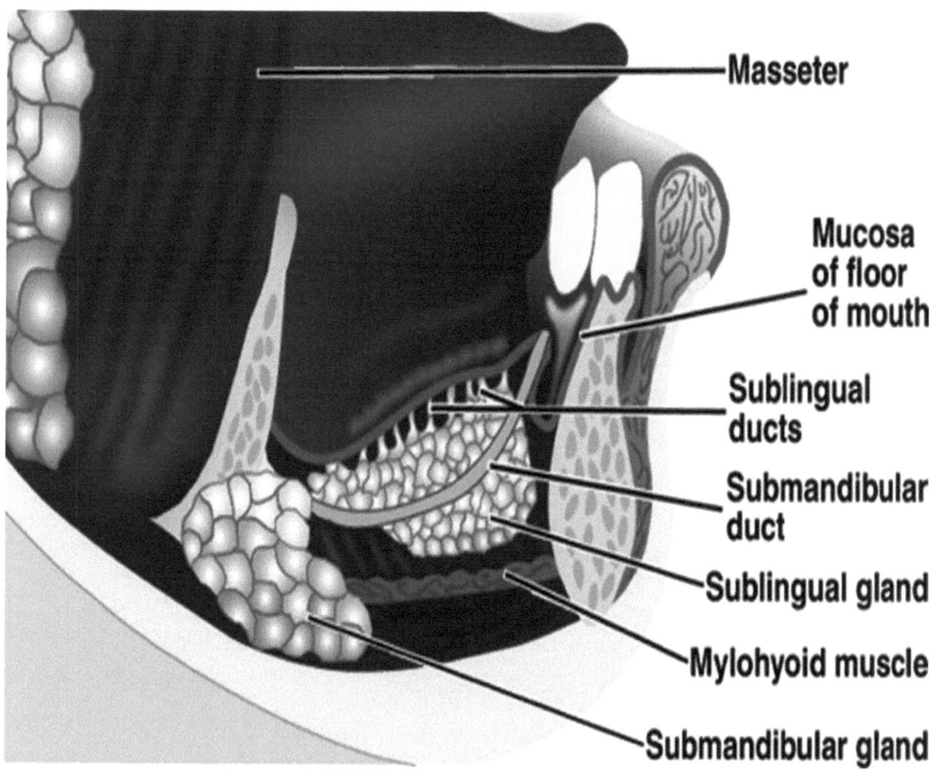

Figure 30. Sublingual gland

Intraperitoneal viscera are:

- ✓ Stomach (except bare area).
- ✓ 2.5 cm at the beginning of the duodenum.
- ✓ Appendix.
- ✓ Cecum (is peritoneal but lacks meso).
- ✓ Colon transverse.
- ✓ Colon sigmoid.
- ✓ Liver (except in the naked area).
- ✓ Pancreas tail.
- ✓ The spleen.
- ✓ Rahm.

Extraperitoneal viscera are:

- ✓ Abdominal esophagus.
- ✓ Duodenum (except 2.5 cm at the beginning).
- ✓ Bare area of the stomach.
- ✓ Ascending colon.
- ✓ Descending colon.
- ✓ Kidneys.
- ✓ Adrenal glands.
- ✓ هاب‌ها.
- ✓ Pancreas (except tail).
- ✓ Bare area of the liver.
- ✓ Aorta.
- ✓ Lower Wisconsin.
- ✓ Bladder.
- ✓ Rectum.

Important peritoneal derivatives are:

- ✓ Greater omentum: Attached to the large curvature of the stomach.

- ✓ Lesser omentum: The small curvature of the stomach and the initial part of the duodenum connects to the liver.
- ✓ Falciform ligament: Attaches the anterior surface of the liver to the posterior surface of the abdominal wall.
- ✓ Round hepatic ligament: Attaches the lower free side of the liver to the umbilicus.
- ✓ Right and left coronary ligaments of the liver: Attaches the upper surface of the liver to the diaphragm.
- ✓ Gastrosplenic ligament: Attaches the stomach to the spleen.
- ✓ Splenural ligament: Attaches the spleen to the left kidney.
- ✓ Gastrocolic ligament: Attaches the stomach to the large intestine.
- ✓ Broad ligament.
- ✓ Ovarian hanging ligament.

Chapter III

Genitourinary System

The urinary tract consists of the following components:

✓ Kidneys.
✓ Bladder.
✓ Urinary tract.

The male reproductive system consists of the following components:

✓ Testicles.
✓ Defender ducts.
✓ Menu bags.
✓ Prostate.
✓ Bulboevertral glands (Cooper).
✓ Penis.

The female external genitalia include the following components:

✓ Ovaries
✓ Uterine tubes
✓ Rahm
✓ Vagina

The female external genitalia include the following components:

✓ Mons pubis.
✓ Large lobbies.
✓ Small lobbies.
✓ Clitoris.
✓ Vulva.
✓ Vestibular glands.

Kidneys (Kidneys or Renes)

Each kidney has 2 levels (anterior and posterior), 2 ends (upper and lower) and 2 sides (internal and external).

The elements passing through the umbilicus of the kidney are (in order from front to back):

- ✓ Renal vein.
- ✓ Renal artery.
- ✓ Renal pelvis.

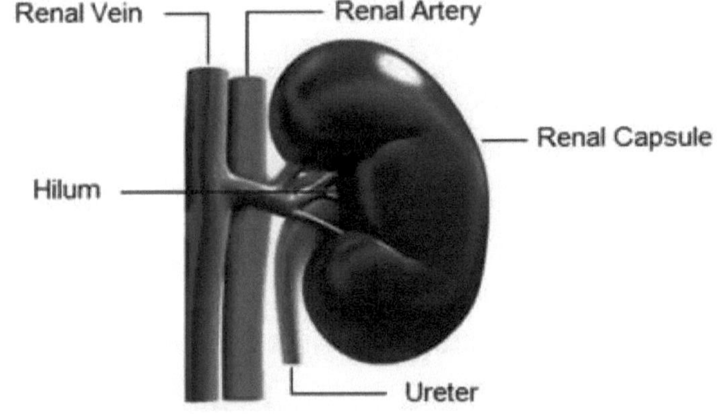

Figure 31. Kidney

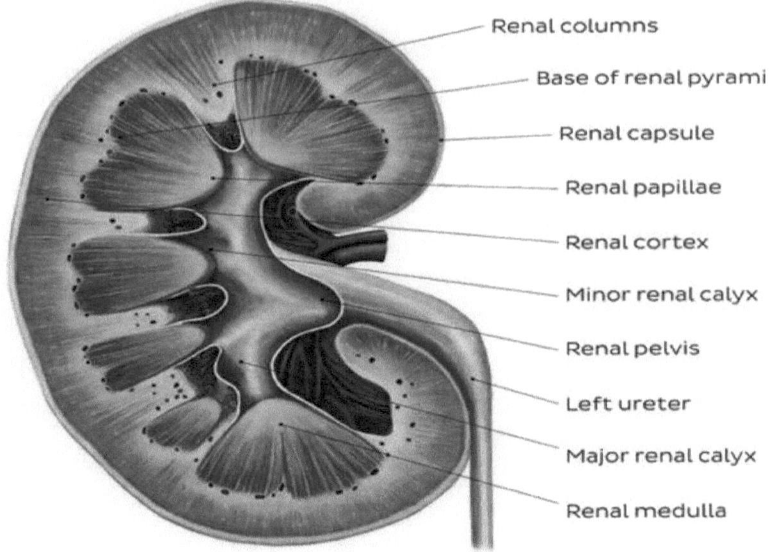

Figure 32. Kidney

- ✓ Due to the presence of the liver on the right side, the right kidney is slightly lower than the left kidney.
- ✓ The right kidney is adjacent to ribs 12 and the left kidney is adjacent to ribs 11 and 12.

Each kidney is surrounded from outside to inside by the following layers:

- ✓ Pararenal fat: This fat is more pronounced on the dorsal surface of the kidney.
- ✓ Renal fascia or Gerota's fascia.
- ✓ Perirenal fat.
- ✓ Fiber capsule.

In a longitudinal section of all 3 main parts can be seen:

- ✓ Cortex
- ✓ Modula: It has 2 parts:

1) Renal Pyramids: They are seen in dark colors. The top of each pyramid is called a papilla. The urine produced in each pyramid is emptied by the papilla into the minor calyx. Each minor calyx receives 1-3 pyramid urine. Every 2-3 minor classes, they empty their urine into a major calyx. The calyces of the major eventually drain urine into the renal pelvis. The renal pelvis is eventually located along the ureter.

2) Renal column: are clearly visible.

Renal sinus: Contains adipose tissue and arteries and nerves that enter the kidney.

- ✓ Each renal pyramid, along with its superficial cortex, is called a renal lobe.
- ✓ Each kidney has 5 segments.
- ✓ The kidneys are extraperitoneal.

Kidney arteries and nerves

- ✓ Renal artery: A branch of the aorta. The right renal artery is longer than the left renal artery and passes behind the inferior vena cava. Each renal artery is divided into 5 branches and each enters one of the renal segments.
- ✓ Renal vein: The renal vein drains directly into the inferior vena cava. The left renal vein is longer and crosses the anterior aorta.
- ✓ Lymph: Discharged to the lumbar nodes.
- ✓ Nerves: Derived from the renal neural network.

Ureters

It transports urine from the kidneys to the bladder.

It has 2 sections:
- ✓ Abdominal part.
- ✓ Pelvic section.

The ureter has 3 narrowing in its path:
- ✓ At the junction with the renal pelvis.
- ✓ At the point of crossing the common iliac artery.
- ✓ At the entrance to the bladder wall.

Urinary bladder

The apex of the bladder connects to the oracle duct.

The lowest part of the bladder is called the bladder neck, which is the most stable part.

When the bladder is empty, two types of mucus can be seen on the inner surface of the bladder:
- ✓ Wrinkled area: These folds are lost during bladder dilation.
- ✓ Trigon smooth area: This area is located in the posterior wall of the inner surface of the bladder. It has 3 heads; Its upper apex is where the ureters enter the bladder, and its lower apex is the beginning of the urethra. Near the lower apex is a bulge called the uvula.

The smooth muscle of the bladder wall is called the detrusor muscle. This smooth muscle around the neck of the bladder forms the internal urethral sphincter (involuntary sphincter).

In men, the upper surface and upper surface of the base of the bladder are covered by the peritoneum; But in women, only the upper surface of the bladder is covered by the peritoneum.

Posterior proximity of the base of the bladder:

✓ In men: rectum, menu bags and vas deferens.

✓ In women: vagina.

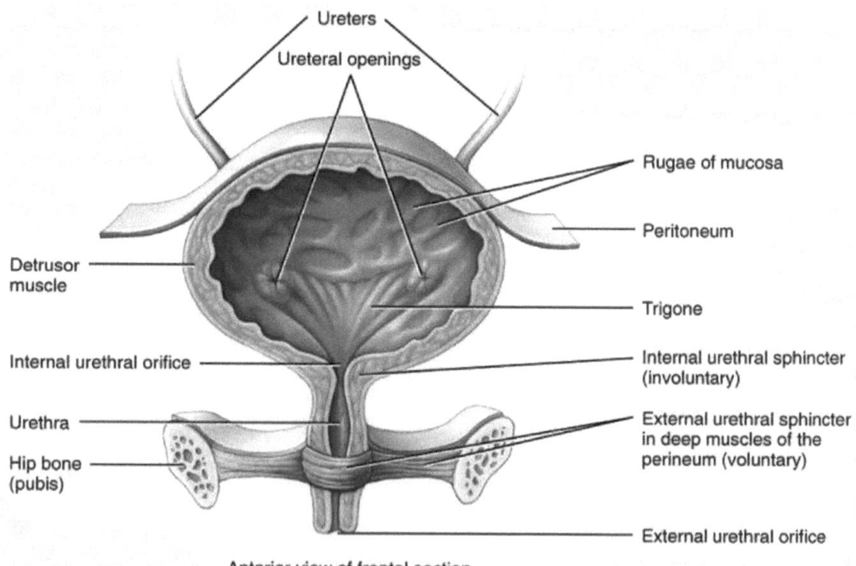

Figure 33. **Urinary bladder**

Bladder arteries and nerves

- ✓ The bladder draws blood from the branches of the internal iliac artery.
- ✓ There is a rich venous network around the bladder.
- ✓ Lymph: It drains into the internal and external iliac lymph nodes.
- ✓ Nerves: originates from the lower hypogastric network.

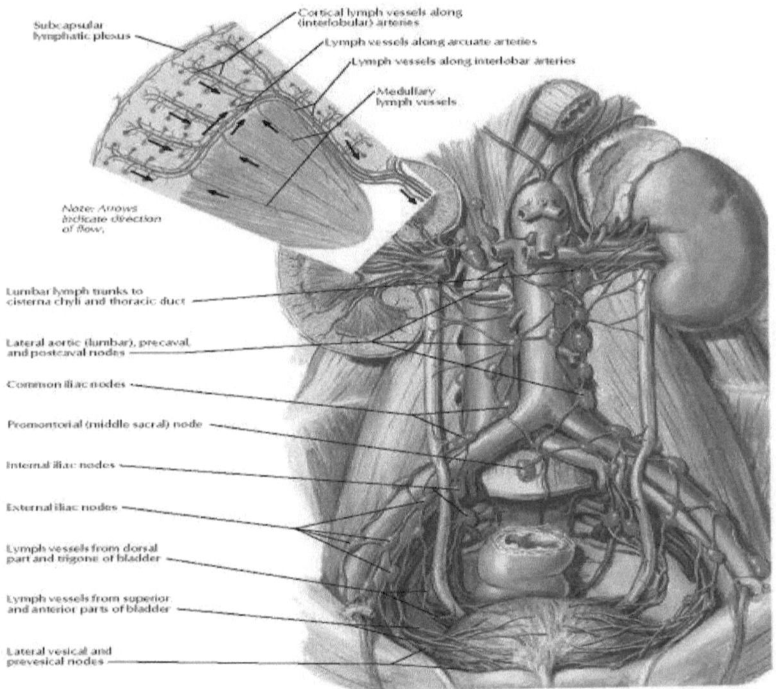

Figure 34. Bladder arteries and nerves

Urethra

The urethra died

It transports urine from the bladder to the outside of the body. It has four sections:

- ✓ Preprostatic section: 1 cm long. It extends from the neck of the bladder to the upper surface of the prostate.

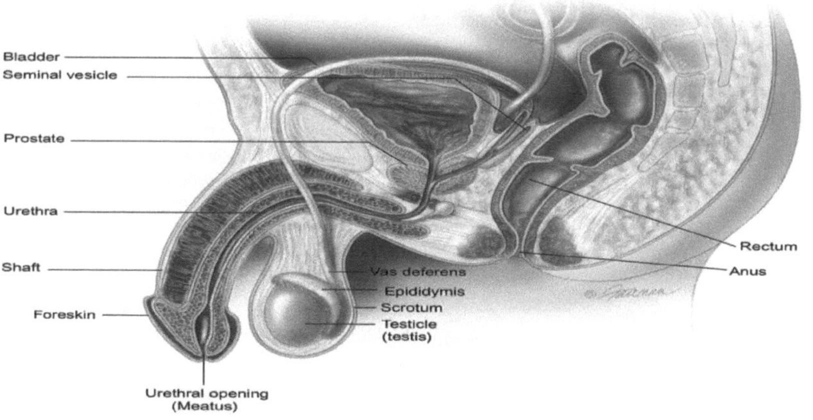

Figure 35. Urethra

Prostate section:

- ✓ It is 4 cm long and is located in the thickness of the prostate gland.
- ✓ It is more expandable than other parts of the urethra.
- ✓ In its posterior wall, there is a urethral crest.
- ✓ On either side of the urethra is the prostate sinus, to which the secretions of the prostate gland drain.
- ✓ In the middle of the urethral ridge is a protrusion called the seminal colliculus, at the apex of which there is a hole that opens into a thick hole in the prostate gland called the utricle. Ejaculatory ducts drain into the lower-lateral part of this hole.

Membranous section:

- ✓ It is approximately 1.5 cm long and is located in the thickness of the urogenital diaphragm.
- ✓ It has the smallest diameter compared to other parts of the urethra.
- ✓ This part of the urethra is surrounded by the external urethral sphincter (voluntary sphincter).

Penis or sponge part:

- ✓ It is about 15 cm long and is located in the thickness of the penis.
- ✓ The secretions of the two bulbovertral glands (Cooper glands) are discharged at the beginning of this section.
- ✓ The urethra is drained into this area.

Female urethra

- ✓ It is 4 cm long.
- ✓ It is located in front of the vagina and parallel to it.
- ✓ The paravertebral glands drain into it.

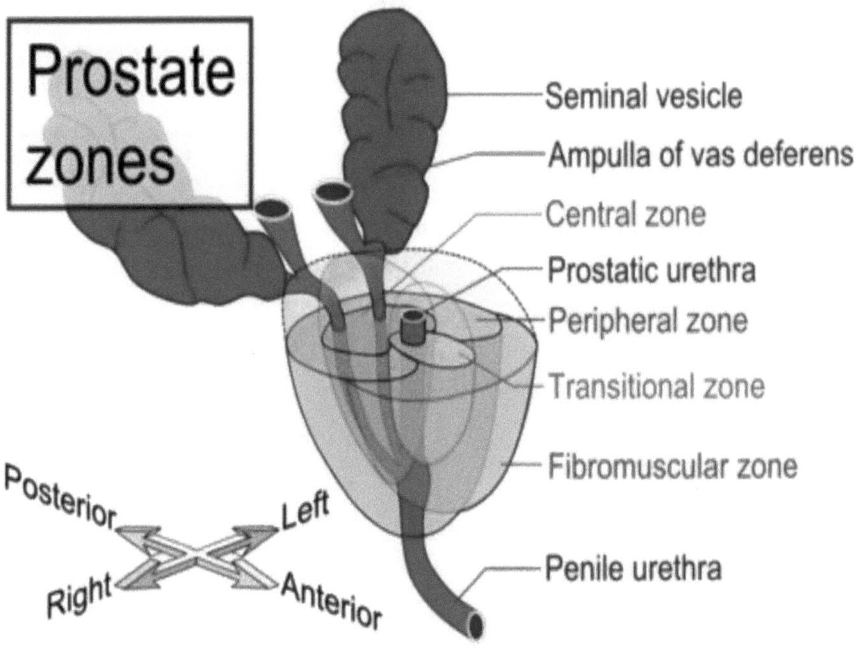

Figure 36. Prostate section:

Testes
- ✓ The testicles are located in the scrotum.
- ✓ The left testicle is slightly lower than the right testicle.
- ✓ The testicle is surrounded from outside to inside by 3 coverings:
1) Tunica vaginalis: It is a peritoneum and consists of two layers of wall and viscera (attached to the testicle). The space between the two is fluid. Tonica vaginalis does not cover the posterior surface of the testis.
2) Tunica albuginea: From this layer, leaflets pass inward and divide the testicle into several lobules. Inside each lobule are seminiferous tubules.
3) Tunica vasculosa.
- ✓ The muscle in the thickness of the scrotal skin is called the dartus.

Epididymis

The twisted tube is 6 meters long and is located behind the testicle. The epididymis is responsible for storing sperm.

It has 3 sections:
- ✓ Head.
- ✓ Body.
- ✓ Tail: It is located along the vas deferens.

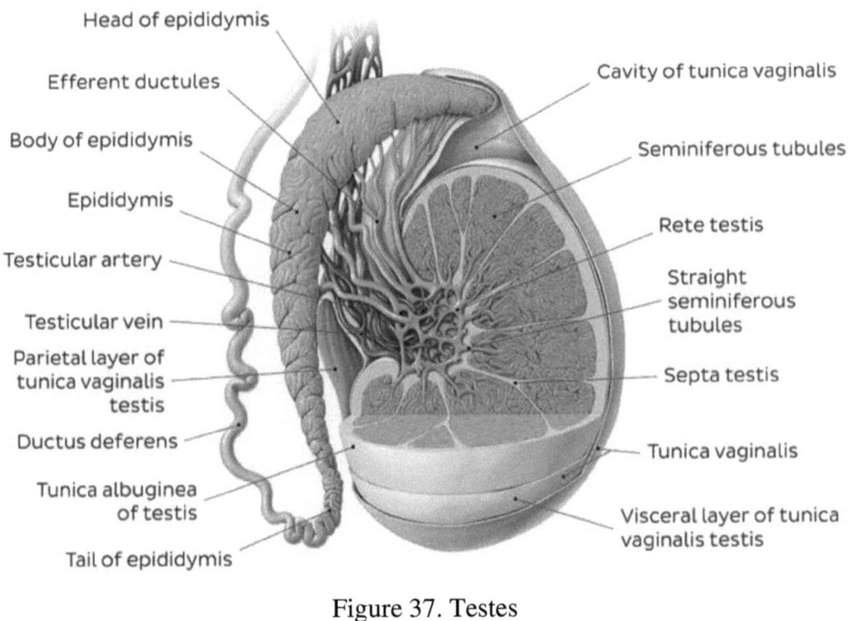

Figure 37. Testes

Ductus deferens

It starts at the tail of the epididymis and, passing through the inguinal canal, enters the pelvis and reaches the back of the bladder, where it dilates, which is called the vas deferens. At this point, the meniscus duct connects to it and forms the ejaculatory duct. The ejaculate passes through the thickness of the prostate and eventually drains into the prostatic urethra.

Menu bags (Seminal vesicles)

✓ There are a pair of secretory glands behind the bladder that are outside the vas deferens.

✓ Most of the semen is secreted by these glands.

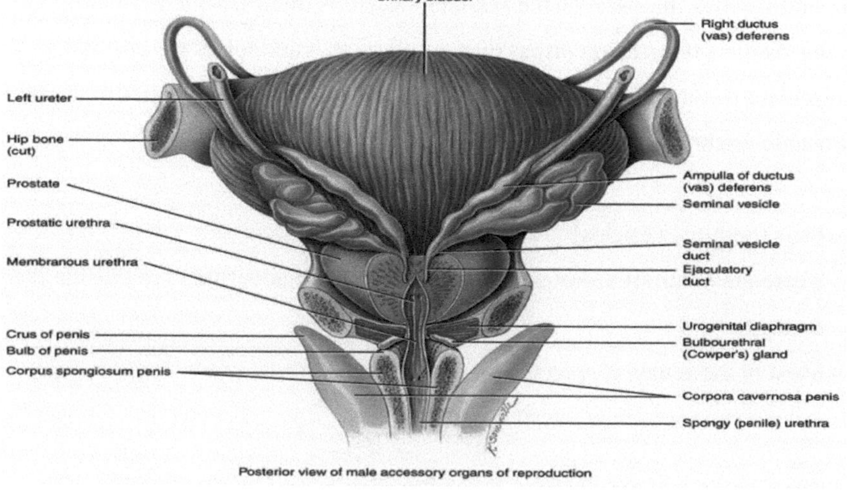

Figure 38. Ductus deferens

Prostate gland

✓ It is located at the bottom of the bladder and above the urogenital diaphragm.

✓ It is adjacent to the rectal ampule from behind.

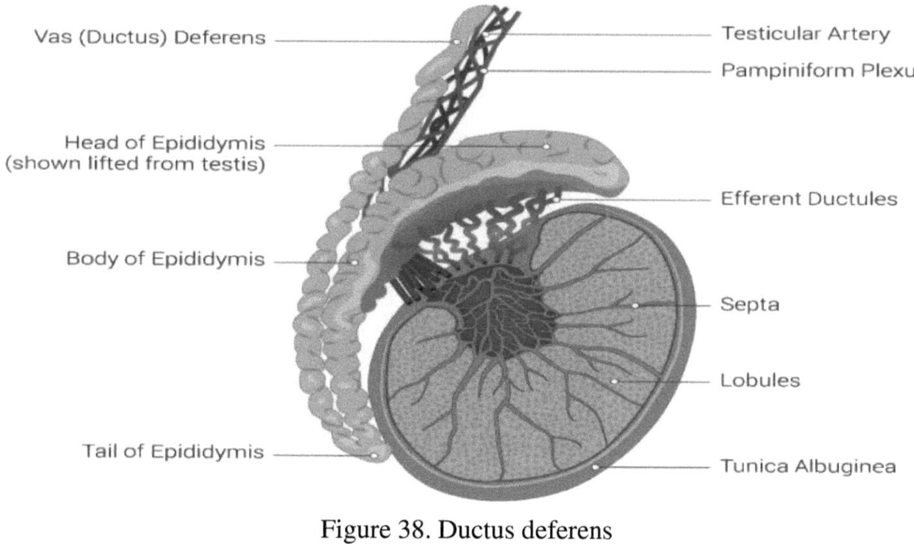

Figure 39. Prostate gland

Bulboevertral glands (Cooper)

- ✓ They are a pair of glands located in the thickness of the urethral-genital diaphragm.
- ✓ It discharges its secretions to the beginning of the spongy urethra.

Prostate vessels and nerves, meniscus sacs, bulbourethral glands and vas deferens

- ✓ Their blood supply is to the arteries of the lower bladder.
- ✓ The nerves are supplied by the hypogastric network.

Penis

There are 3 objects in its thickness; Each of these objects is surrounded by tonica albugine:

- ✓ 2 cave body (Corpus cavernosum).
- ✓ 1 Sponge body (Corpus spongiosum): In its thickness, the urethra of the penis passes.

The penis has 3 parts:

1) Root: The root of the penis consists of 3 parts:
   - ✓ 2 Columns (Crus): The posterior part of the cave objects. The columns are covered by the ischemic cavernous muscle. Each column connects to the ischiopubic arch of the pelvis.
   - ✓ 1 Bulb: The posterior part of the body is spongy. The bubble is covered by the muscle of the bulbospongius.
2) Body.
3) Head: The head of the penis is called Glans. Glans is made up of a spongy body. The skin on the penis is called the prepuce, which is connected to the abdominal surface of the penis by a skin fold called the frenulum.

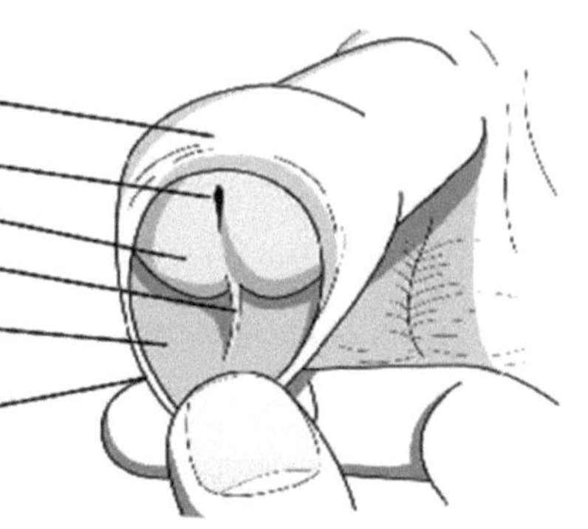

Figure 40. Penis

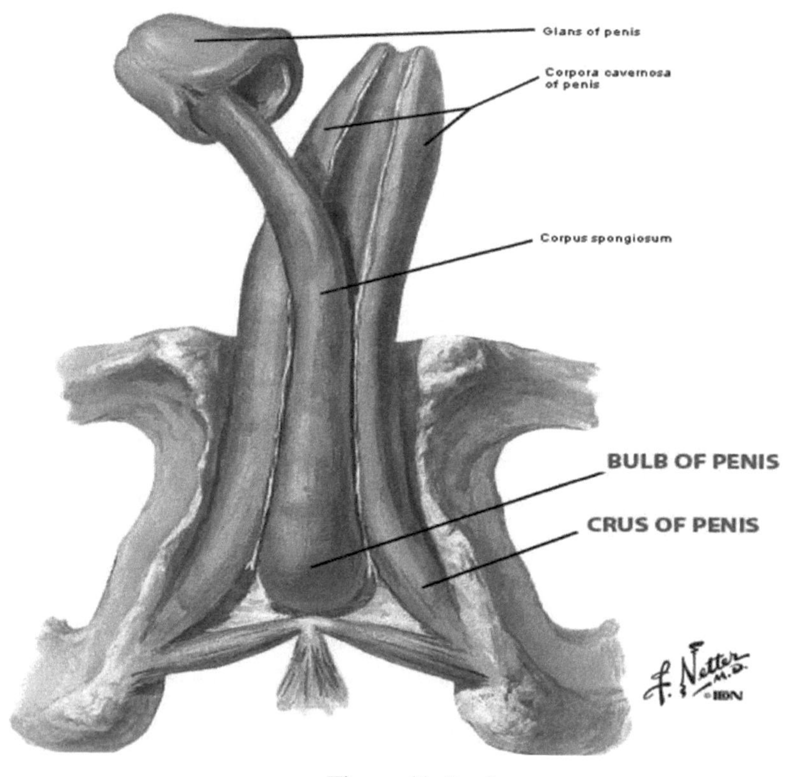

Figure 41. Penis

Blood vessels and nerves of the penis

- ✓ Blood flow to the penis is provided by the internal pudendal artery (a branch of the internal iliac artery).
- ✓ Deep vein blood drains into the venous network around the penis.
- ✓ The nerves of the penis are supplied by the pudendal nerve.

Ovaries

- ✓ It is a pair of gonads that are attached to the posterior surface of the uterine ligament on each side.
- ✓ The inner surface of the ovary is covered with fallopian tubes.
- ✓ The upper pole of the ovary is adjacent to the fallopian tube.
- ✓ The lower pole of the ovary is connected to the uterus by the ovarian ligament.

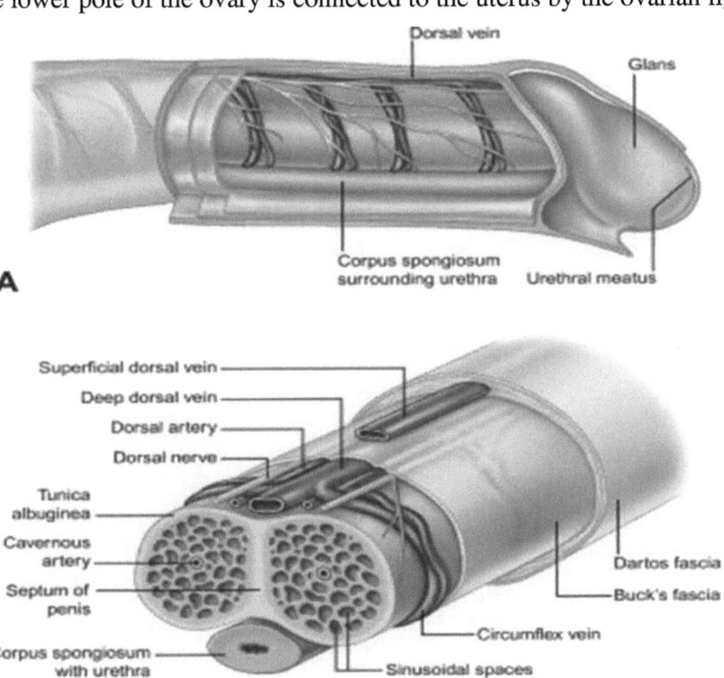

Figure 42. Blood vessels and nerves of the penis

Ovarian arteries and nerves

- ✓ Arteries: Ovarian arteries (a branch of the descending aorta).
- ✓ Veins: The left ovarian vein flows into the left renal vein and the right ovarian vein into the inferior vena cava.
- ✓ Nerves: Provided by the ovarian network.

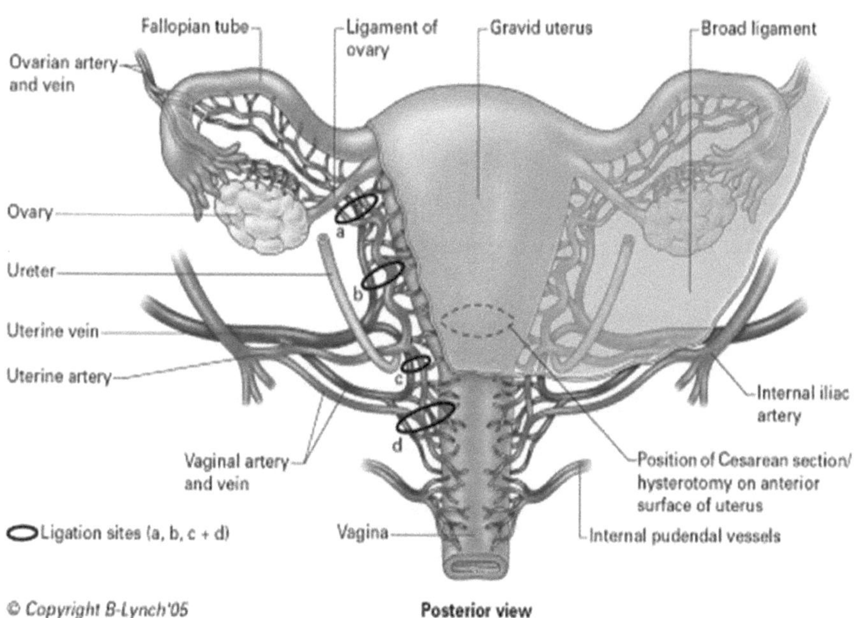

Figure 43. Ovarian arteries and nerves

Uterine tubes

It is 10 cm long and extends from the uterus to the ovary.

The fallopian tube consists of 4 sections (respectively from outside to inside):

- ✓ Infandibulum: It has filaments on its edge called fimbriae that are adjacent to the ovary. The fimbriae are responsible for processing the released egg from the ovary and transferring it into the fallopian tube.

- ✓ Ampoule: The largest and widest part of the fallopian tube. Fertilization takes place in this area.
- ✓ Isthmus (Strait): It has a thick wall.
- ✓ Intramural (inner wall): The part of the fallopian tube that is the thickness of the uterine wall.

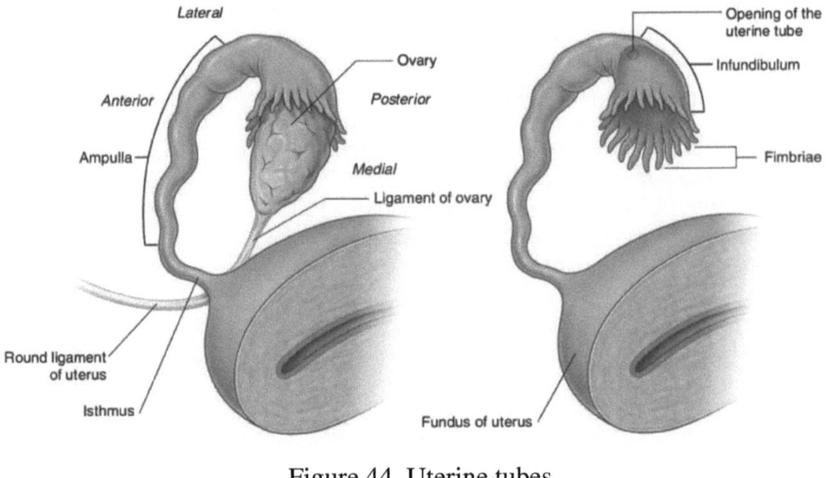

Figure 44. Uterine tubes

Tubular arteries and nerves

- ✓ The blood supply to the fallopian tubes is responsible for the ovaries and uterine arteries.
- ✓ Nerves: Supplied from hypogastric and ovarian networks.

Uterus

The wall of the uterus consists of 3 layers (respectively from outside to inside):

- ✓ Perimetrium: A membrane of visceral peritoneum.
- ✓ Myometrium: It is muscular.
- ✓ Endometrium: The lining of the mucosa.

The uterus is generally divided into two parts:
- ✓ The body of the uterus: It is the moving part of the uterus and forms the upper two thirds of the uterus. The upper lateral part of the uterine body is called the uterine horns, to which the fallopian tubes return. The part of the uterine trunk that is located above these holes is called the fundus.
- ✓ Cervix: The cylindrical and fixed part of the uterus. It has 2 holes:
  1) Internal os: It leads to the uterine cavity.
  2) External os: It enters the vagina.

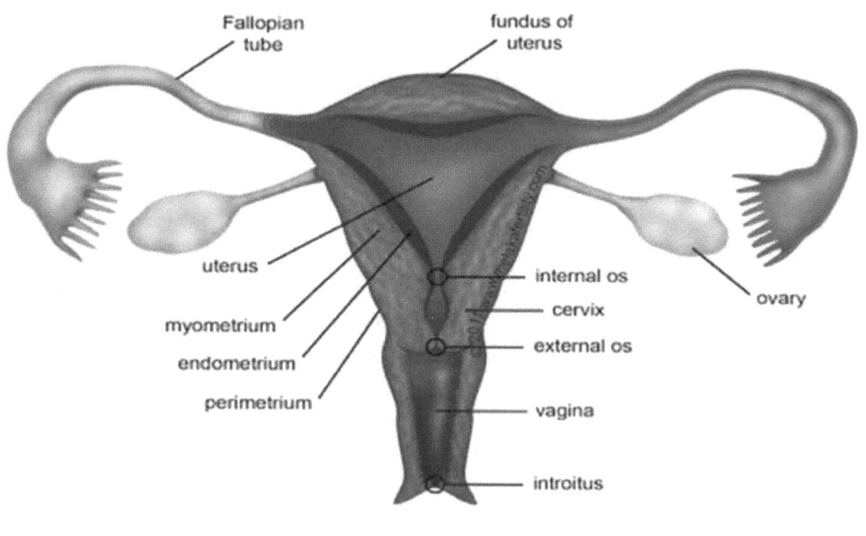

Figure 45. Uterus

Some of the uterine ligaments are:
- ✓ Broad Ligament: It is made of peritoneum and after enclosing the uterus, it connects both sides of the uterus to the pelvic wall.
- ✓ Suspensory ligament of the ovary: It is a peritoneum. It is connected to the upper pole of the ovary and through it the ovarian vessels pass through.
- ✓ Ovarian ligament: The lower pole of the ovary connects to the side of the uterus.
- ✓ Round ligament: Attaches the side of the uterus to the labia majora.

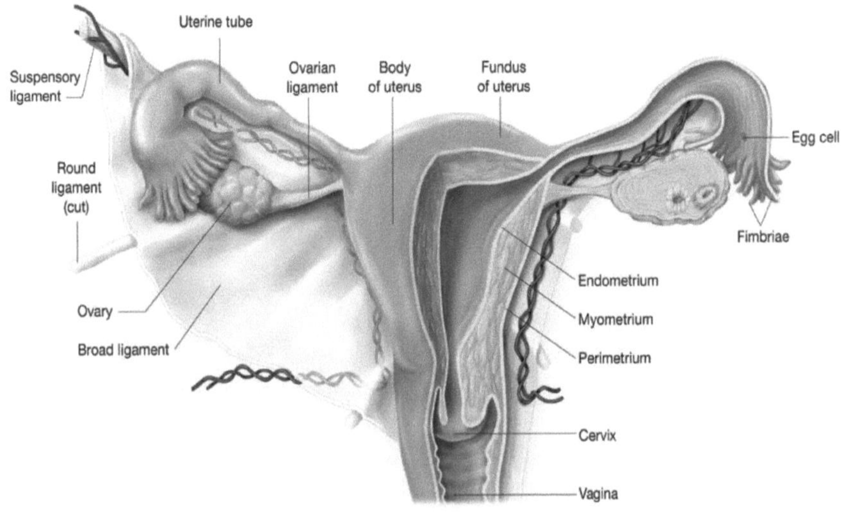

Figure 46. uterine ligaments

Tip

✓ The round ligament, ovarian ligament and fallopian tubes are located in the thickness of the broad uterine ligament.

✓ The peritoneal junction that forms between the uterus and the rectum (Rectouterine or Douglas junction) is considered to be the lowest part of the peritoneal cavity.

The factors that protect the uterus are:

✓ Uterine ligaments.

✓ Pelvic diaphragm (anal and coccygeal muscles).

✓ The curved position of the front of the uterus relative to the vagina.

Adjacent to the uterus are:

✓ From the front and bottom: bladder.

✓ From behind: rectum and small intestinal arches.

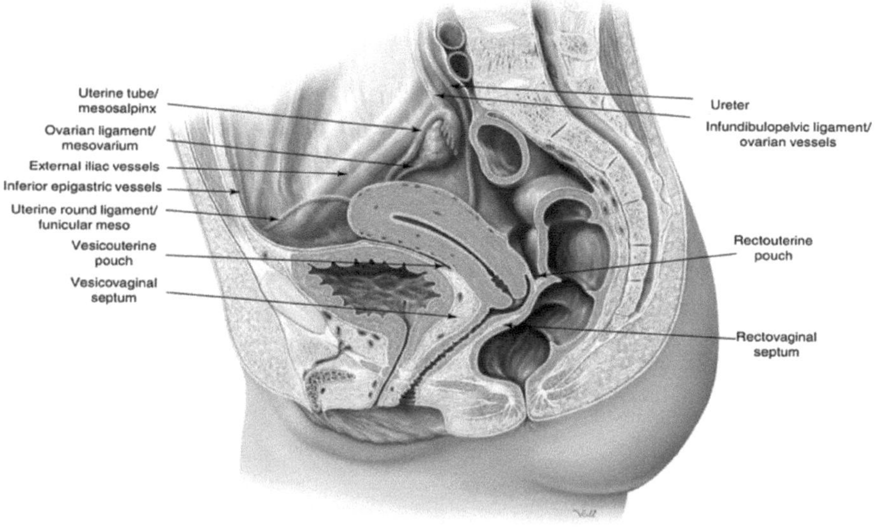

Figure 47. Adjacent to the uterus

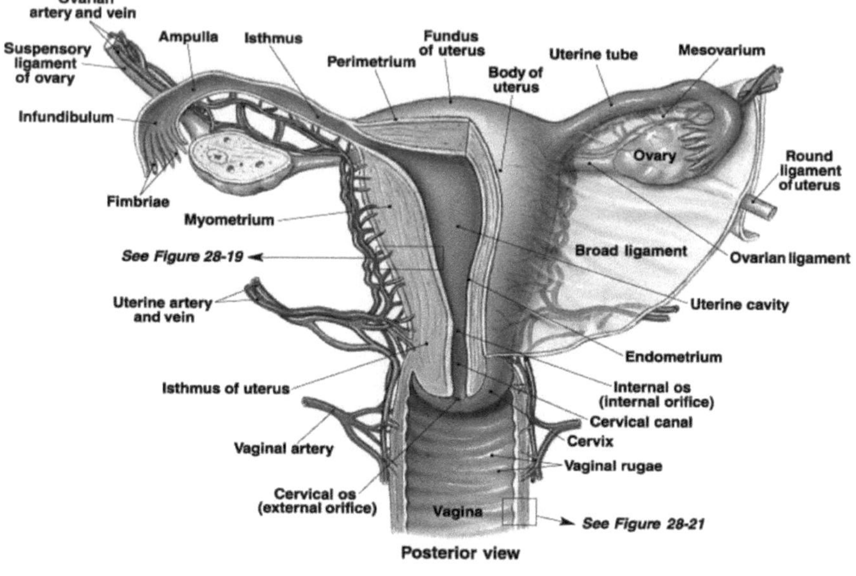

Figure 48. Adjacent to the uterus

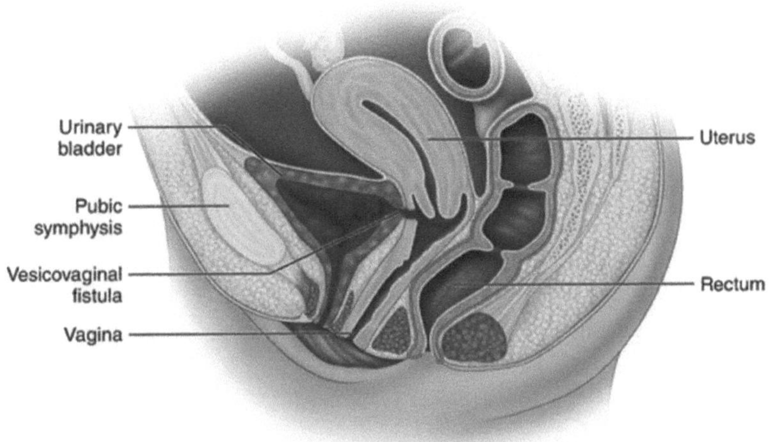

Figure 49. Adjacent to the uterus

Uterine arteries and nerves

- ✓ Uterine blood supply is responsible for the uterine artery (a branch of the internal iliac artery).
- ✓ The uterine vein drains into the internal iliac vein.
- ✓ Nerves: Supplied from the lower hypogastric network.

Vagina

- ✓ The length of the posterior wall is 9 cm and the length of the anterior wall is 7.5 cm.
- ✓ The space between the vaginal wall and the cervix is called the Fornix. There are 4 types of fornix (anterior, posterior, right and left).

Adjacent to the vagina are:

- ✓ From the front: the base of the bladder and urethra.
- ✓ From behind: rectum and anal canal.
- ✓ Lateral Proximity: Lifting muscle of the anus and ureter.

The outer opening of the vagina is covered by a membrane called the hymen. This veil is torn during the first sexual intercourse.

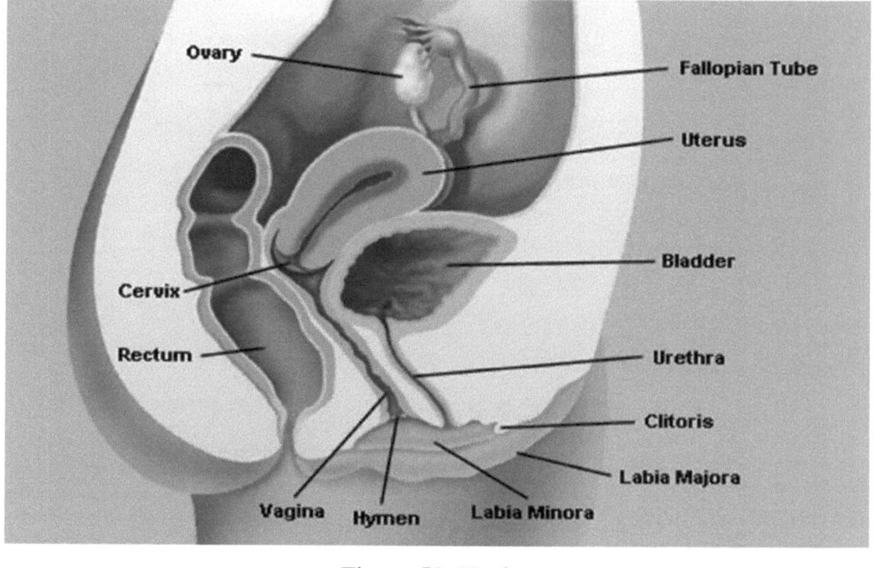

Figure 50. Vagina

Vaginal arteries and nerves
- ✓ Artery: The vaginal branch of the internal iliac artery.
- ✓ Nerves: Lower and sacral hypogastric networks.

Mons pubis
- ✓ The bulge contains fat that can be felt and seen in front of the symphysis pubis.
- ✓ In the adult it is covered by hair.

Large labia (Labium majors)
- ✓ There are two large folds of skin.
- ✓ The two folds are connected from the anterior and posterior by the anterior and posterior interface, respectively.

Labium minors

The space between the small lobes is called the vulva.

The following holes open into the valve space. (In order from top to bottom):

- ✓ Urethral hole.
- ✓ Paravertral duct interventions.
- ✓ Vagina.
- ✓ Involvement of large vestibular ducts.

The skin on the clitoris and the clitoris phrenolum are formed by the anterior connection of the small lobes to each other.

Clitoris

It is equivalent to a penis in men and has an erectile effect due to the entry of cave objects in their thickness.

It has 3 sections:

- ✓ Root.
- ✓ Body
- ✓ Head

Bulb of vestibule: Located on either side of the vagina and has an erectile function.

They are covered by the muscles of the bulbospongius.

The head of the clitoris is located at the anterior end of the small labia.

Greater vestibular glands

- ✓ They are located behind the vestibular bubbles.
- ✓ It is covered by the muscle of the bulbospongius.
- ✓ The ducts of these glands drain on either side of the vaginal opening.

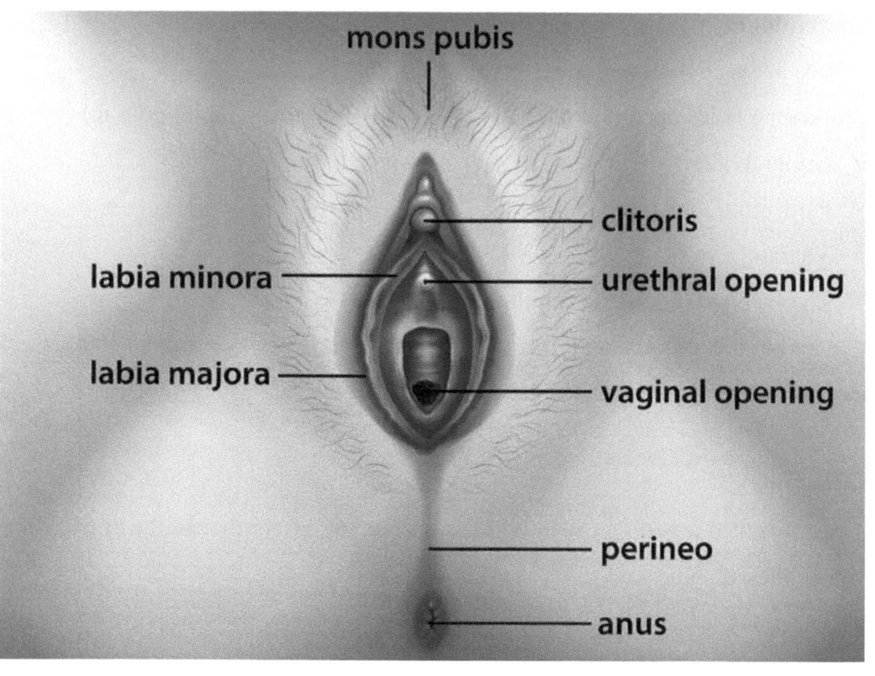

Figure 51. Clitoris

Perineum

It is a rhombus-shaped space between two thighs.

This rhombus-shaped space can be divided into two triangles:

- ✓ Anterior Triangle (Urinary-Genital Triangle): Includes scrotum, penile root, and female external genitalia. The triangle itself is divided into superficial and deep spaces by a membrane called the perineal membrane.
- ✓ Posterior triangle (anal triangle): Includes the anus. This triangle has right and left ischemic cavities. Inside these cavities is fat.

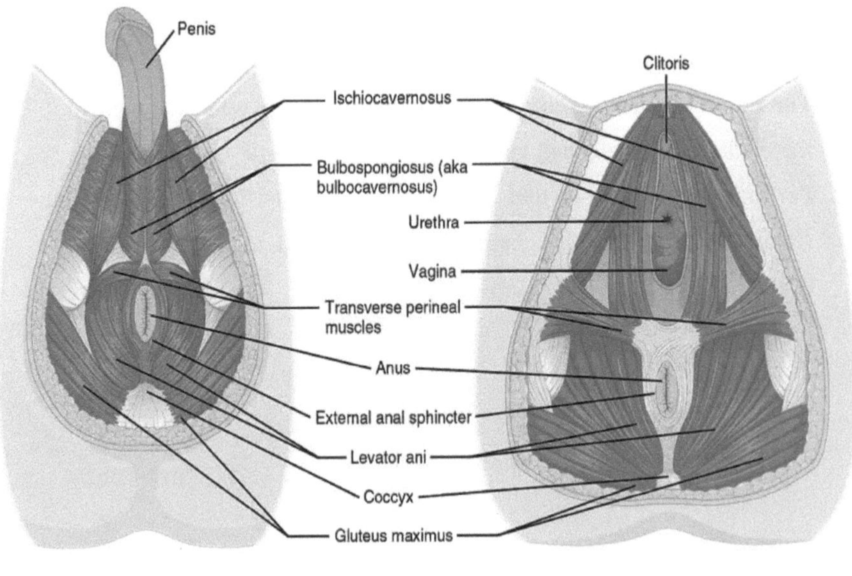

Figure 52. Perineum

Golden Tips of the Season

✓ The elements passing through the umbilicus of the lung are (in order from front to back):

1) Renal vein

2) Renal artery

3) Renal pelvis

✓ Due to the presence of the liver on the right side, the right kidney is slightly lower than the left kidney.

✓ The right kidney is adjacent to ribs 12 and the left kidney is adjacent to ribs 11 and 12.

✓ Each renal pyramid, along with its superficial cortex, is called a renal lobe.

✓ Each kidney has 5 segments.

✓ The kidneys are extraperitoneal.

- ✓ The ampulla is the largest and widest part of the fallopian tube. Fertilization occurs in this area.
- ✓ The round ligament, ovarian ligament and fallopian tubes are located in the thickness of the broad uterine ligament.
- ✓ Peritoneal obstruction that forms between the uterus and rectum (Rectouterine or Douglas obstruction). It is considered as the lowest part of the peritoneal cavity.

Chapter IV

Endocrine Device

Hypophysis

Inside the cavity of the Turkish saddle (Sela thoraca) is the sphenoid bone.

The pituitary gland is connected to the hypothalamus above.

It has 2 main lobes:

- ✓ Anterior lobe (adenohypophysis).
- ✓ Posterior lobe (neurohypophysis).

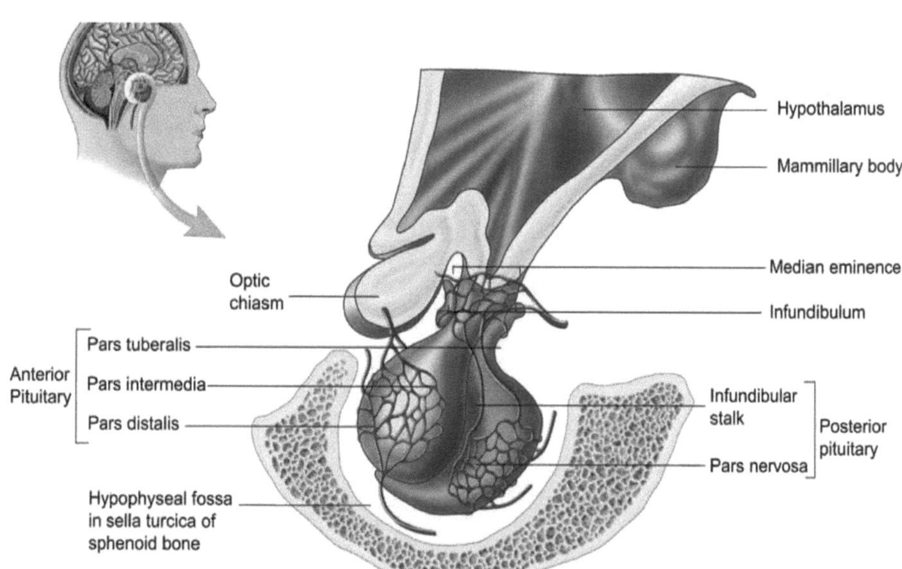

Figure 53. pituitary gland

Pineal gland

- ✓ It is located above and between the upper ridges of the midbrain.
- ✓ It secretes hormones such as melatonin.

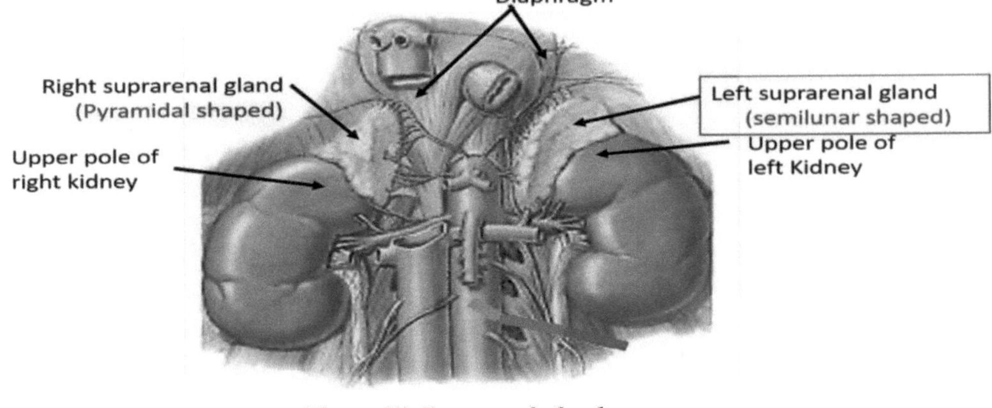

Figure 54. Pineal gland

Suprarenal glands

- ✓ The adrenal glands are located above and in front of the upper pole of the kidneys. A fascia sheet separates the adrenal gland from the kidneys.
- ✓ The right adrenal gland is triangular and the left adrenal gland is crescent-shaped.
- ✓ It has 2 parts, cortex and medulla.

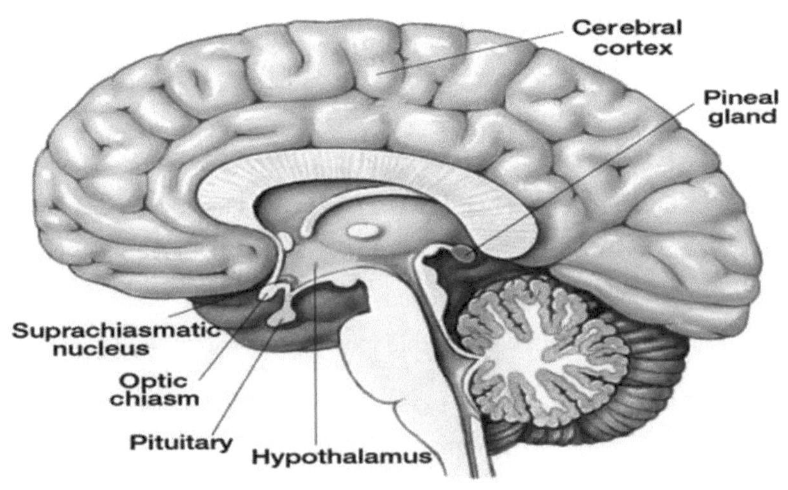

Figure 55. Suprarenal glands

Thyroid gland and parathyroid glands

✓ The thyroid gland is located in the neck area and surrounds the anterior and lateral surface of part of the trachea.

✓ The thyroid gland has two lobes, the right and the left, which are connected by a part called the Isthmus; Isthmus is located in front of the second and third rings of the trachea.

✓ A capsule of connective tissue surrounds the thyroid gland.

✓ On the posterior surface of each thyroid lobe are two parathyroid glands.

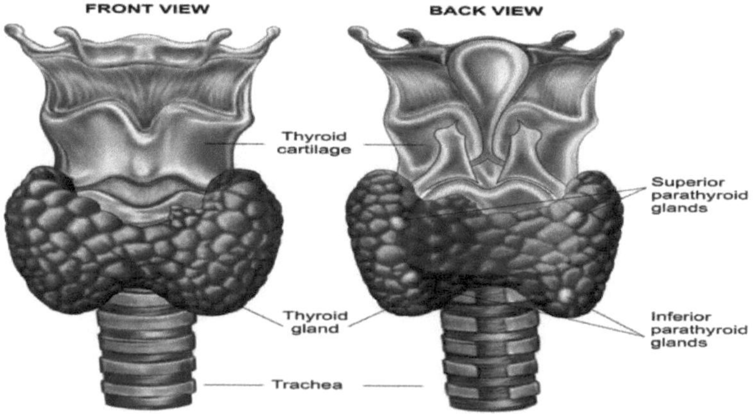

Figure 56. Thyroid gland

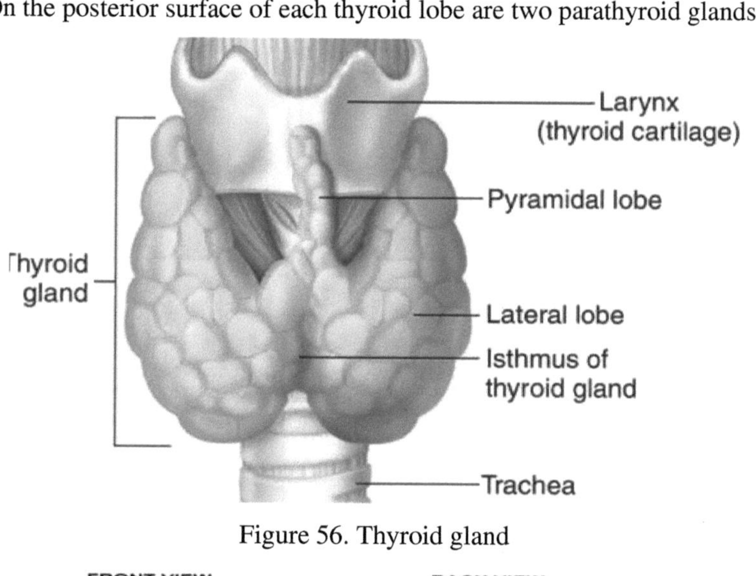

Figure 57. Thyroid gland

Thyroid blood supply is responsible for 2 arteries:

✓ Upper thyroid: A branch of the external carotid artery

✓ Lower Thyroid: A branch of the thyroid cervical trunk (a branch of the subclavian artery). This artery is adjacent to the laryngeal recurrent nerve.

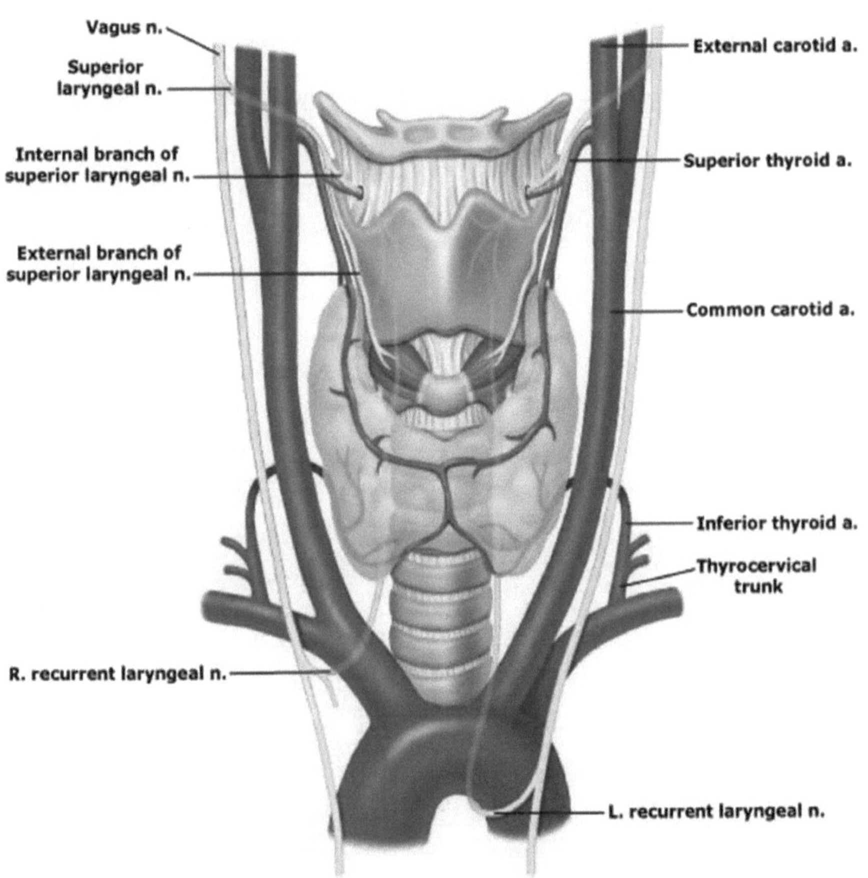

Figure 58. Thyroid blood supply is responsible for 2 arteries

- ✓ Pituitary circulation is of the portal system type.
- ✓ The right adrenal gland is triangular and the left adrenal gland is crescent-shaped.
- ✓ The isthmus of the thyroid gland is located in front of the second and third rings of the trachea.
- ✓ The inferior thyroid artery is adjacent to the laryngeal recurrent nerve.

Chapter V

Eyes and Ears

Eye

Eye ball

- ✓ The eyeball is covered by the Tenon's Capsule, except in the anterior.
- ✓ The wall of the eyeball consists of 3 layers. (In order from outside to inside):
- ✓ Fibrous layer: It has 2 parts

1) Anterior one-sixth: It is clear and colorless and is called Cornea.

2) Sixth posterior: It is white and is called sclera.

Vascular layer: It has 3 sections (in order from front to back):

1) Iris: A broad ring with a pupil in the center. The base of the iris is attached to the ciliary body. Eye color is due to the presence of pigments in the iris. It has 2 types of annular muscles (pupil constrictor) and radial muscle (pupil dilator).

2) Ciliary body: Attaches to the iris base from the front and to the choroid from the back. It has 3 levels (anterior, external and internal). The inner surface has two parts: anterior (uneven) and posterior (smooth); The anterior part of the inner surface has appendages and valleys between these appendages. Zonular fibers attach to these areas; The other side of these fibers attaches to the lens capsule of the eye. The contraction of the smooth muscles of the ciliary body causes the zonular fibers to loosen, resulting in the convexity of the lens of the eye. (Adaptation process).

3) Choroids: From the back of the eyeball to the back of the ciliary body.

✓ The iris annular muscle is innervated by the parasympathetic fibers of the third pair of cerebral nerves and the iris radial muscle is innervated by the sympathetic nerves.

✓ The muscles of the ciliary body are innervated by the parasympathetic fibers of the third pair of nerves.

Neural layer or Retina: It has 2 parts:

1) Anterior part: No visual receptor.

2) Posterior part: has a visual receptor. At the back of this section is an area called the macula lutea, the center of which is sunken and called the central cavity (Fovea Centralis); This area has the maximum visual sensitivity. 3 mm inside the yellow spot is the optic disk, which lacks a visual receptor and is called the blind spot. The optic nerve from this area leaves the eyeball.

✓ The junction of the visual and non-visual part of the retina is called the serrated circle (Ora serrata).

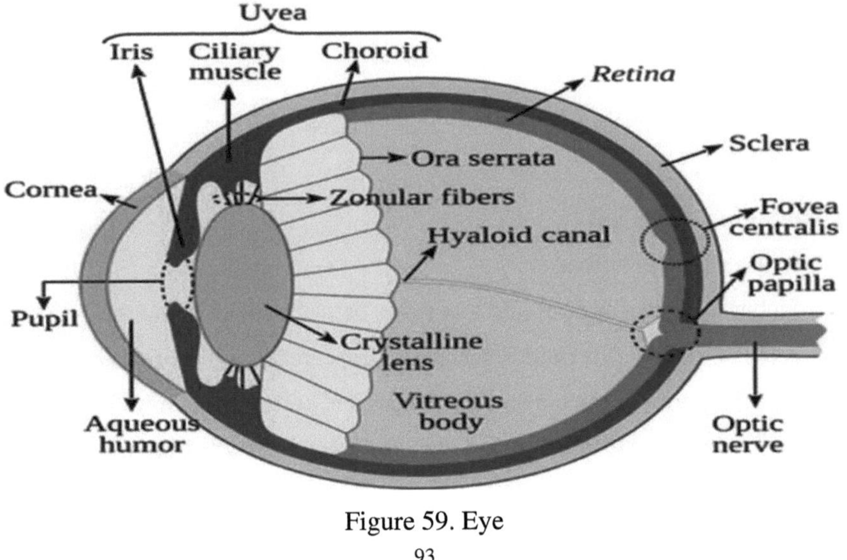

Figure 59. Eye

Conjunctive

It is a clear, vascular membrane that covers the inner surface of the eyelids and the anterior part of the sclera (continues at the periphery of the cornea as the corneal epithelium); Therefore, the conjunctiva has 2 parts:

✓ Eyelid section

✓ The eyeball parts

Between these two parts is the conjunctival end (Fornix Conjunctiva); Dead ends are divided into two types, upper and lower.

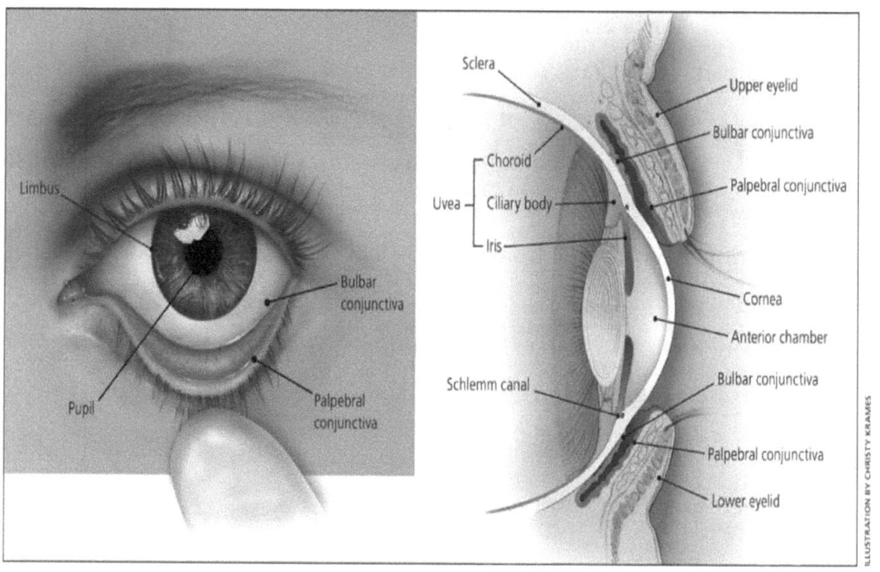

Figure 60. Conjunctive

The contents of the eyeball

The contents of the eyeball are:

✓ Aqueous humor: A clear liquid that flows between the lens and the cornea. The process of making this fluid is such that it is secreted into the posterior chamber by the capillaries of the ciliary appendages and enters the anterior chamber after passing through the pupil hole. This fluid is eventually reabsorbed into the sludge channel.

✓ The space between the anterior surface of the lens and the posterior surface of the cornea is divided by the iris into two parts. (These two spaces are connected to each other by the pupil):

1) Anterior chamber: The space between the iris and the cornea.

2) Posterior chamber: The space between the iris and the lens.

✓ Lens: The lens of the eye is oval (convex on both sides) and is surrounded by a capsule. The lens is attached to the ciliary bodies by xenular fibers. The posterior surface of the lens is more convex.

✓ Viterous body: It is a clear jelly and fills the space between the posterior surface of the lens to the retina. The vitreous retains the shape of the eyeball.

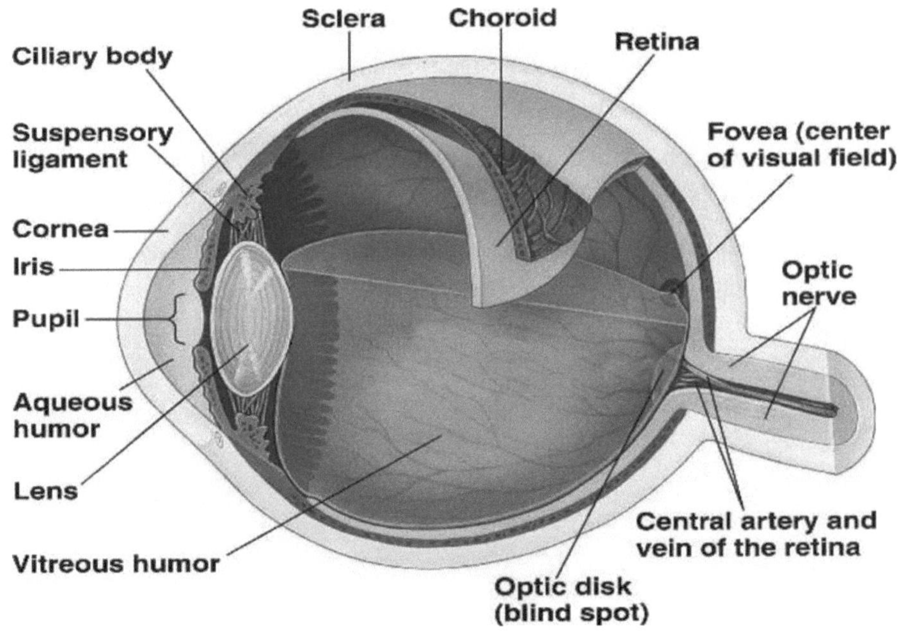

Figure 61. Lens

Tip

✓ The lens and cornea lack capillaries and are nourished by the aqueous humor.

Eyelids or palpebrae

The upper eyelid is larger and more mobile than the lower eyelid.

Eyelid cleft: The distance between the upper and lower eyelids

The inner end of the eyelid cleft is called the medial canthus and the outer end is called the lateral canthus. The inner canthus has the following anatomical features:

✓ Lacrimal lake.

✓ Crescent (Plica semilunaris).

✓ Lacrimal caruncle.

✓ Lacrimal papilla: There is a free edge at the inner end of each eyelid, and at the top is a hole called the lacrimal punctum.

At the thickness of each eyelid is a fibrous plate called the tarsus. The free edge of the eyeballs is located on the free side of the eyelid, and the other end is connected to the edges of the eyeball by another fibrous membrane called the orbital septum.

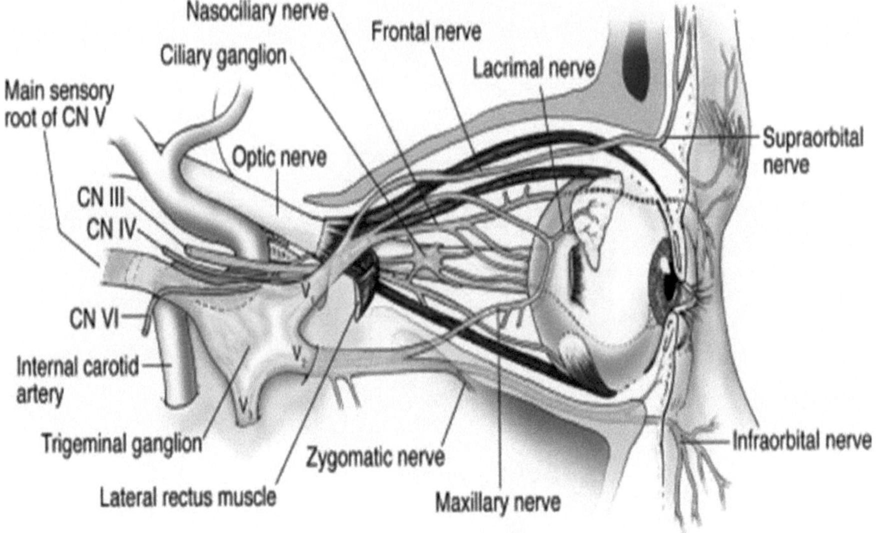

Figure 62. Eyelids or palpebrae

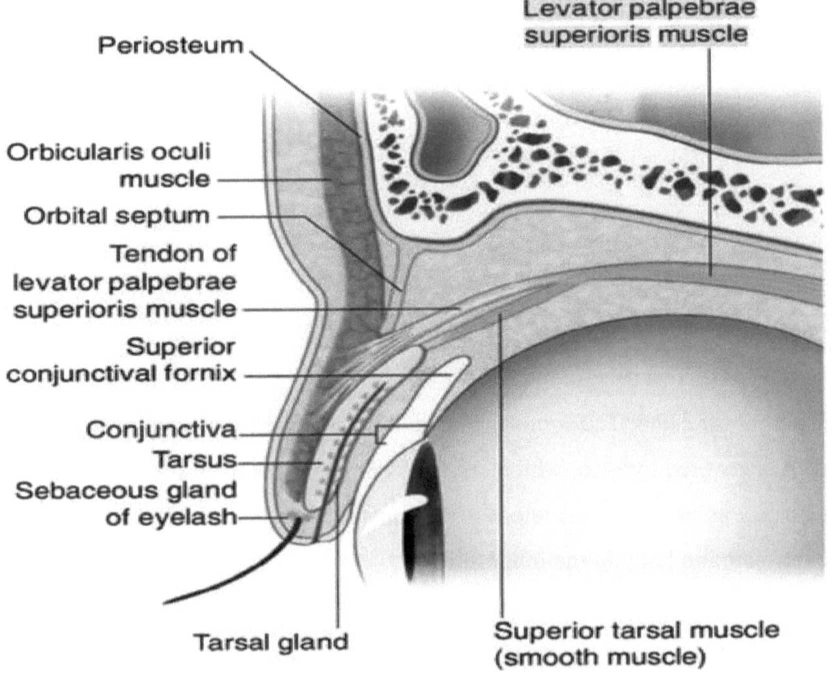

Figure 65. Arteries and nerves of the eye

Ear

The ear is divided into 3 areas:

- ✓ Outer ear.
- ✓ Middle ear.
- ✓ Inner ear.

Outer ear

It has 2 sections:

- ✓ Earlobe: Has a cartilaginous structure.
- ✓ External ear canal: The sounds collected by the earlobe direct the ear canal. The duct is covered by skin, which contains cerumen glands in the thickness of the skin in this area. The skeleton of this duct is cartilaginous in one third of the outer part and bony in the inner third.

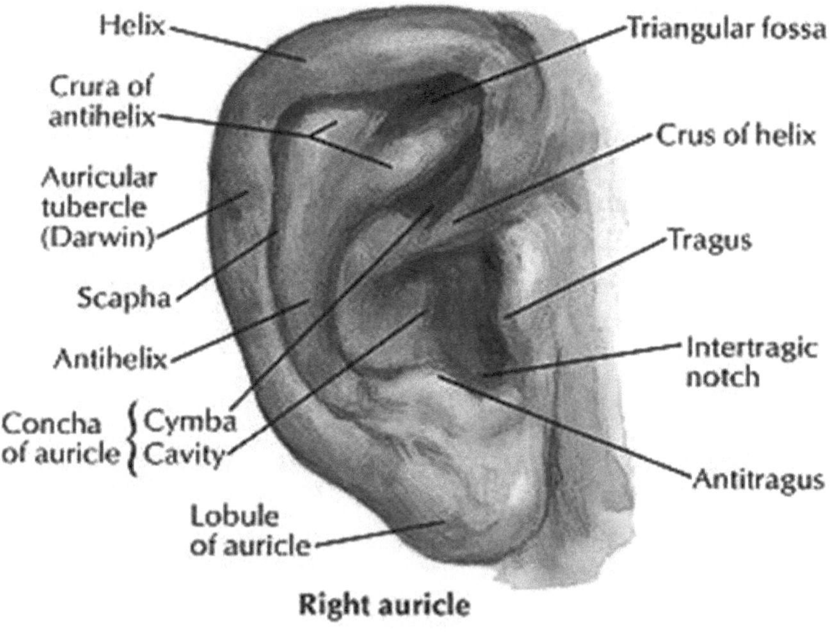

Figure 66. Ear

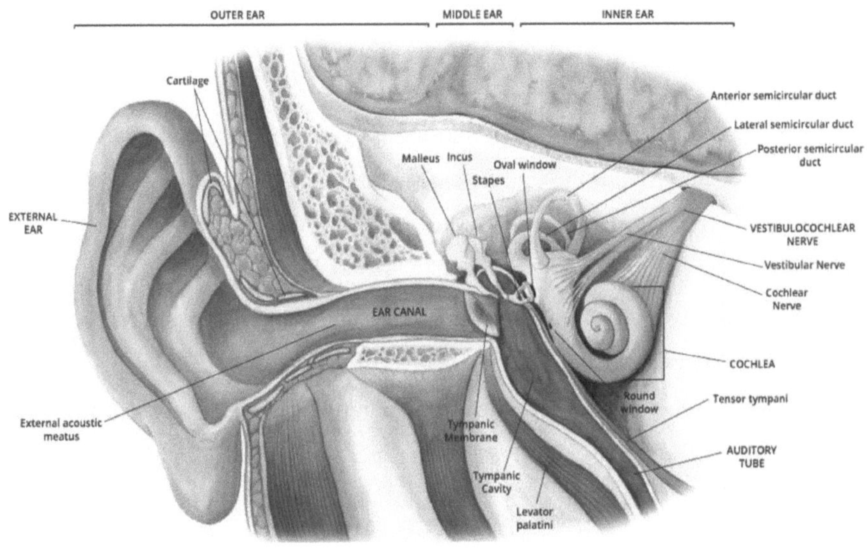

Figure 67. Ear

Middle ear or tympanic cavity

The walls of the middle ear are:

- ✓ Upper wall: Tegment tympani of the temporal bone.
- ✓ Bottom wall: The bony part of the jugular cavity.
- ✓ Exterior wall: eardrum.

Interior wall: The 3 most important structures in an interior wall are:

- ✓ Promontary: A bulge created by the first cochlear arch.
- ✓ Oval or Vestibular window: Blocked by the base of the stapes. This window is between the middle ear and the vestibular space of the inner ear.
- ✓ Cochlear or Round window: Blocked by a curtain called the secondary tympanic membrane. This membrane is a barrier between the middle ear and the tympanic cochlea of the inner ear.

Posterior wall: The two most important structures in the posterior wall are:

- ✓ Aditus: A window that connects the middle ear to the mastoid cavities.

✓ Pyramidal protrusion: At the top of this protrusion is a hole for the exit of the stapes muscle tendon.

✓ The eustachian tube connects the middle ear to the nasopharynx. The posterior third (from the middle ear) is bony and the anterior two thirds (from the pharynx) are cartilaginous.

Anterior wall: The two most important structures in the anterior wall are:

✓ Tympanic tensor muscle duct.

✓ Eustachian tube (ear canal): The eustachian tube connects the middle ear to the nasopharynx.

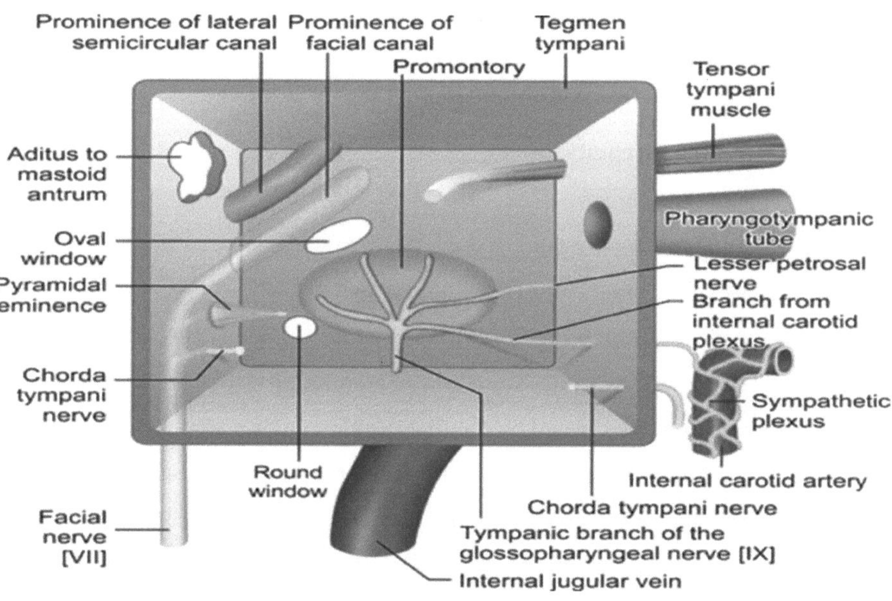

Figure 68. Middle ear or tympanic cavity

The contents of the middle ear are:

- ✓ Ear bones:

1) Hammer (Malleus): Attaches to the eardrum.

2) Indus (Incus).

3) Stapedus: Its base is attached to the oval window.

4) Ligaments.

Middle ear muscles:

- ✓ Tensor tympani muscle: It is innervated by the trigeminal nerve (pair V).

- ✓ Stapedus muscle: Nerve by the facial nerve (pair VII).

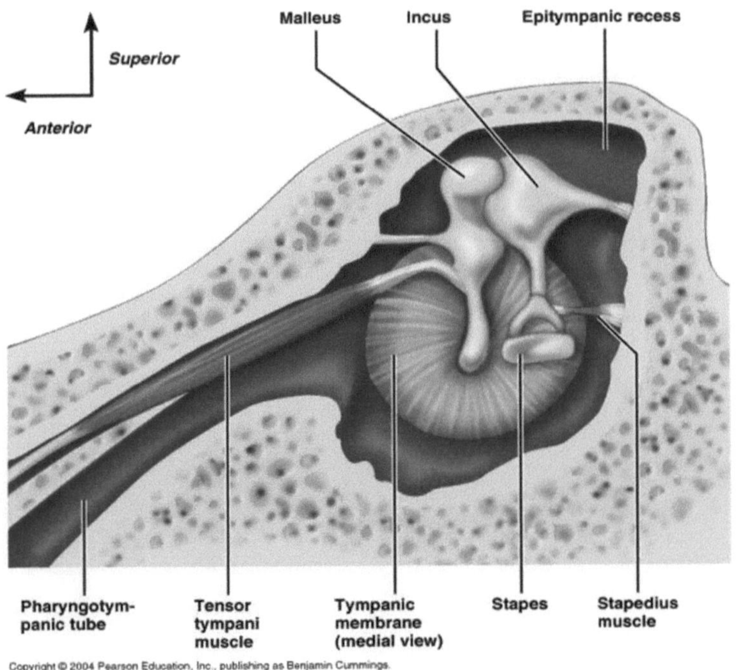

Figure 69. Middle ear muscles

✓ The middle ear and inner ear are located in the thickness of the pterygoid (temporal part) of the temporal bone.

Inner ear (labyrinth)

The inner ear consists of 2 parts:

1) Bone labyrinth (Osseous labyrinth): The bony labyrinth is divided into 3 parts:

✓ Atrium or vestibule: The atrium is located in the middle of the bony labyrinth and connects to the semicircular canals and the cochlea. The vestibule has two holes or valves called the oval window and the round window.

✓ Semicircular canals: semicircular canals are composed of 3 semicircular canals perpendicular to each other, which are named according to their position into 3 types: anterior (upper), lateral and posterior.

✓ Cochlea: The oldest part of the bony labyrinth.

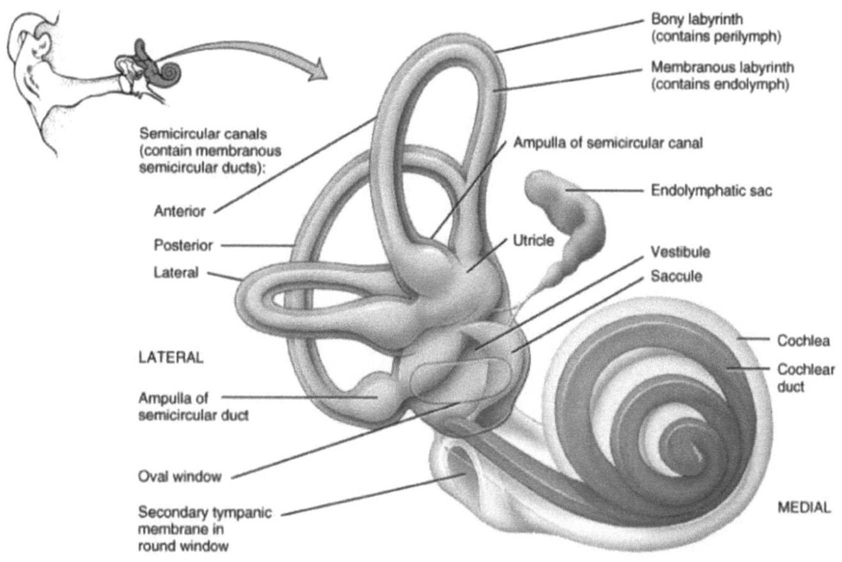

Figure 70. Inner ear (labyrinth)

2) Membranous labyrinth: The membrane labyrinth is located inside the bony labyrinth and almost takes its shape. The membranous labyrinth is located inside the bony labyrinth. Membrane labyrinth has 3 parts:

✓ Cochlear duct: Contains auditory receptors (cortical bodies). In cross section, the spiral duct is triangular in shape and has three walls: upper (Vestibular membrane), lower (Basilar membrane) and outer (Spiral ligament). The lower wall contains auditory receptors (cortical objects).

✓ Utricle and Saccule: These two sacs are located inside the vestibule and contain sensitive balance receptors called macula.

✓ Semicircular canals: One end of each of these canals dilates and forms the ampulla. Inside each ampoule are sensitive balance receptors called Crista.

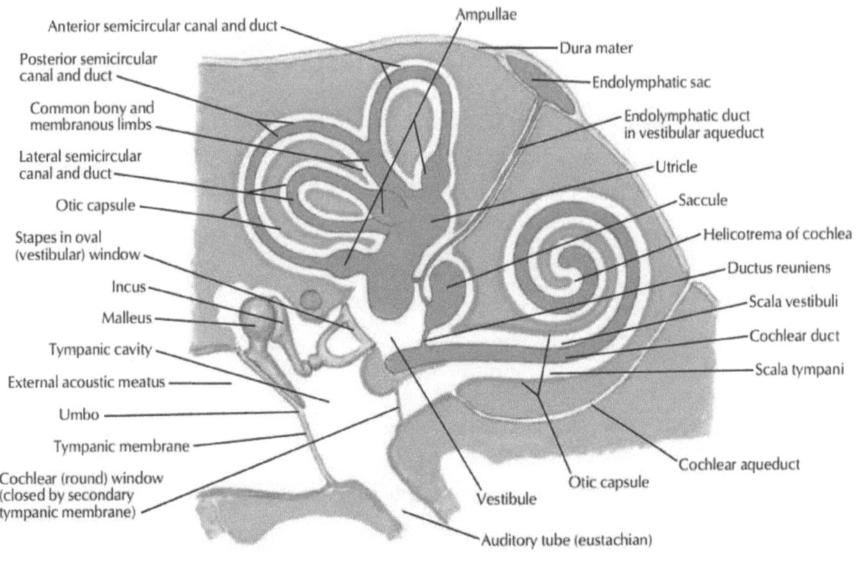

Figure 71. Inner ear (labyrinth)

The space inside the bony labyrinth is divided into two spaces by a spiral ligament and a cochlear duct:

✓ Scala vestibule.

✓ Scala tympani.

The membranous labyrinth is filled with endolymph fluid and the bony labyrinth is filled with perilymph fluid.

The cell body of the auditory receptors is located in the spiral ganglion at the base of the helical bony blade. The axons of these neurons form the auditory part of the balance-auditory nerve.

The nerve fibers of the crystals and macula form the balance part of the auditory balance nerve.

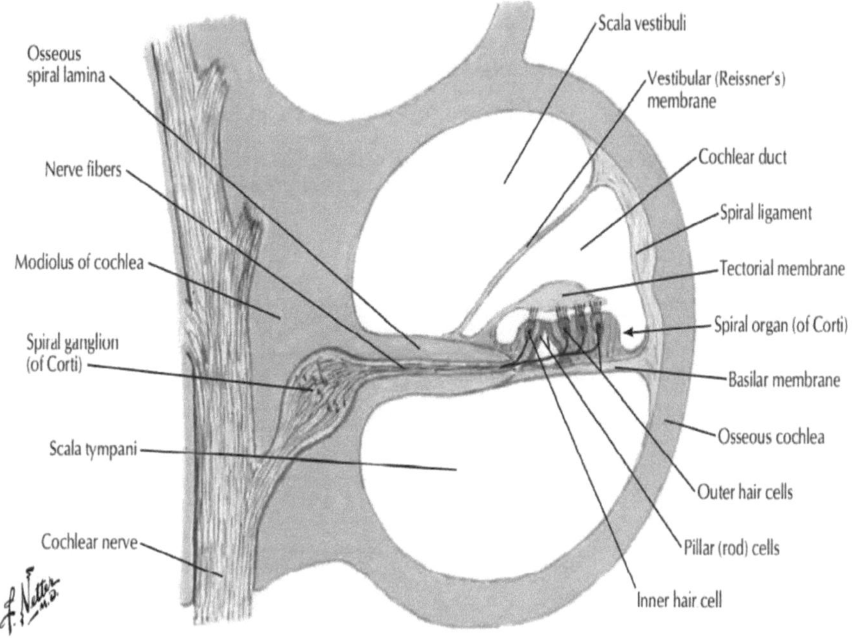

Figure 72. Inner ear (labyrinth)

- ✓ The junction of the cornea with the sclera is called the limbus. In the thickness of this place, there is Schlemm's canal or Sclera venous sinus, the aqueous humor is reabsorbed into this canal.
- ✓ The iris has two types of muscles: annular (pupil constrictor) and radial (pupil dilator).
- ✓ The iris annular muscle is innervated by the parasympathetic fibers of the third pair of cerebral nerves and the iris radial muscle is innervated by the sympathetic nerves.
- ✓ The muscles of the ciliary body are innervated by parasympathetic fibers of the third pair of nerves.
- ✓ The junction of the visual and non-visual part of the retina is called the serrated circle (Ora serrata).
- ✓ Nerves of the external muscles of the eye: Nerves III, IV and VI of the brain.
- ✓ The general sensation of the eyeball is transmitted by the ophthalmic nerve (a branch of the V cerebral nerve).
- ✓ The sense of sight is directed through the cerebral nerve II (optic nerve).
- ✓ The external ear canal is cartilaginous in one third of the external third and bony in the inner two thirds.

- ✓ The walls of the middle ear are:
1) Upper wall: Tegment tympani of the temporal bone
2) Bottom wall: The bony part of the jugular cavity
3) Exterior wall: eardrum
4) Inner wall:
   - ✓ Nose (Promontary).
   - ✓ Oval or Vestibular window.
   - ✓ Cochlear or Round window.

5) Posterior wall:
- Aditus.
- Pyramidal bulge.

6) Anterior wall:
- The tympanic tensor muscle duct.
- Eustachian tube opening (ear canal).
- The Eustachian tube connects the middle ear to the nasopharynx. The posterior third (from the middle ear) is bony and the anterior two thirds (from the nose) are cartilaginous.
- The middle ear and inner ear are located in the thickness of the temporal bone.
- The membranous labyrinth is filled with endolymph fluid and the bony labyrinth is filled with perilymph fluid.

References

Gray's Anatomy

Anatomy of Snell

Moore's Anatomy

Anatomy of Zubota

Clinical Anatomy

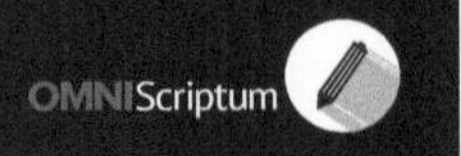

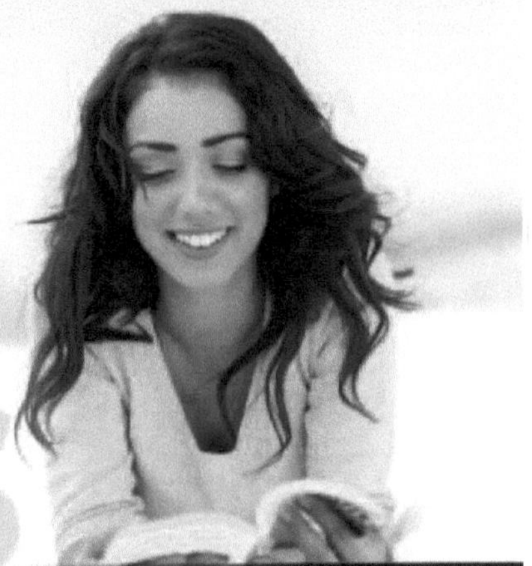

Buy your books fast and straightforward online - at one of world's fastest growing online book stores! Environmentally sound due to Print-on-Demand technologies.

Buy your books online at
www.morebooks.shop

Kaufen Sie Ihre Bücher schnell und unkompliziert online – auf einer der am schnellsten wachsenden Buchhandelsplattformen weltweit! Dank Print-On-Demand umwelt- und ressourcenschonend produziert.

Bücher schneller online kaufen
www.morebooks.shop